MOSBY
An affiliate of Elsevier Science

ISBN 0-7234- 3314-3

First published 2003
Reprinted 2003

Cataloguing in Publication Data
Catalogue records for this book are available from the US Library of
Congress and British Library.

Note
Medical knowledge is constantly changing. As new information becomes
available, changes in treatment, procedures, equipment and the use of
drugs become necessary. The authors and publishers have, as far as it is
possible, taken care to ensure that the information given in this text is
accurate and up to date. However, readers are strongly advised to confirm that the information, especially with regard to drug usage, complies
with latest legislation and standards of practice.

ELSEVIER SCIENCE your source for books,
journals and multimedia
in the health sciences
www.elsevierhealth.com

The
publisher's
policy is to use
**paper manufactured
from sustainable forests**

Printed by Grafos S.A. Arte sobre papel, Spain.

Acknowledgements

For Eleanor and Henry, and for Alexa and Lauren

To our wives Katie and Devra, for their understanding, grace and tolerance.

Preface

Rheumatic diseases are common and account for a significant proportion of consultations in primary care.[1] The most common reason for referral or consultation is back pain, although soft tissue rheumatism and osteoarthritis (OA) also contribute to a considerable workload (Figure 1). Nearly all middle-aged and elderly people have some degree of OA.[2] Inflammatory joint diseases are less prevalent but the nature of these conditions often leads to a significant workload, especially when there is a shared care approach with a specialist centre. Rheumatoid arthritis (RA) affects more than 1% of the population[3] and there is a similar prevalence of the different sero-negative spondyloarthritides. The metabolic joint diseases, particularly gout, are also common.[4]

The diagnosis of most rheumatic diseases is made from a history and clinical examination, and is a skill that is learned from experience. Investigations should be undertaken to confirm a diagnosis, rather than for "screening", as the results will often be misleading. There are no short cuts to the diagnosis that will reduce the need for clinical assessment. Unfortunately, education at either undergraduate or postgraduate level for primary care physicians on aspects of rheumatic diseases is often inadequate. We did not intend to write a comprehensive textbook of rheumatology, but hope to offer some practical guidance on the diagnosis and management of common conditions that could be undertaken without the need for specialist referral, to offer guidance on referral to secondary care, and to discuss the practical aspects of shared care of inflammatory joint diseases. We also hope this book may be helpful to trainees in rheumatology, and that students of medicine, nursing and professions allied to medicine may find the advice given in this book useful for the management of their patients.

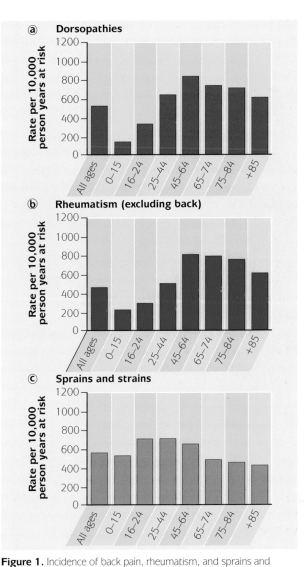

Figure 1. Incidence of back pain, rheumatism, and sprains and strains in general practice in the UK. Reproduced with permission from Linaker CH *et al. Ballieres Clin Rheumatol* 1999; **13**: 197–215

Our aim in this book was to be as didactic as possible whilst attempting to avoid controversy. The sections on the management of polymyalgia rheumatica and gout are purposefully detailed, as these are both inflammatory diseases that are often managed in primary care. It is inevitable that some specialists will have a different opinion on the management of certain conditions and we apologize if this leads to any confusion in management. The advice given in this book is our personal opinion based upon both published data and many years of clinical practice. We hope it provides a useful tool in reducing the burden of these dreadful diseases.

Frank McKenna
Lee Simon
May 2002

Abbreviations

CMC	carpo-metacarpal (joint)
COX	cyclo-oxygenase
coxib	COX-2 inhibitor
CPPD	calcium pyrophosphate crystal deposition disease
CTD	connective tissue disease
DIP	distal interphalangeal (joint)
DMARD	disease-modifying anti-rheumatoid drug
GI	gastrointestinal
MCP	metacarpo-phalangeal (joint)
MI	myocardial infarction
MTP	metatarso-phalangeal (joint)
NSAID	non-steroidal anti-inflammatory drug
OA	osteoarthritis
PAN	polyarteritis nodosa
PIP	proximal interphalangeal (joint)
PMR	polymyalgia rheumatica
PsA	psoriatic arthritis
RA	rheumatoid arthritis
ReA	reactive arthritis
RSI	repetitive strain injury
SLE	systemic lupus erythematosus
SNS	sero-negative spondylo-arthropathy
SSRI	selective serotonin re-uptake inhibitor
TCA	tricyclic antidepressant
TENS	trans-cutaneous electrical stimulation
TNF	tumour necrosis factor

Contents

1003181966

General Principles of Diagnosis

When making a diagnosis of any patient with joint pain, as in other branches of medicine, it is advisable to consider broad categories rather than specific diseases. A careful history should lead to a confident differential diagnosis that can be confirmed from clinical examination and simple investigations.

Joint pain can be characterized as either:

(a)   soft tissue rheumatism or

(b)   arthritis,

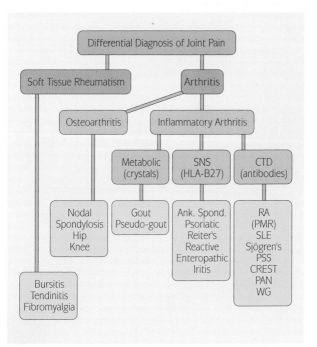

Figure 2. Differential diagnosis of joint pain. CTD, connective tissue disease; PAN, polyarteritis nodosa; PMR, polymyalgia rheumatica; PSS, systemic sclerosis; RA, rheumatoid arthritis; SLE, systemic lupus erythematosus; SNS, sero-negative spondylo-arthropathy; WG, Wegener's granulomatosis.

and arthritis as either:

(a) OA or

(b) inflammatory arthritis.

Inflammatory arthritis should be considered as three groups of diseases:

(a) connective tissue diseases (associated with auto-antibodies, e.g. RA or lupus);

(b) sero-negative spondylo-arthritides (associated with HLA-B27, e.g. psoriatic arthritis or ankylosing spondylitis);

(c) metabolic arthritis (associated with crystals, e.g. gout or pseudo-gout).

A mental framework as shown in Figure 2 should be used as an "aide-mémoire" *in history taking.*

History taking

In order to differentiate arthritis from soft tissue rheumatism, and OA from inflammatory arthritis, we need to consider:

1. The pattern of joint symptoms.

2. Any history of joint swelling.

3. The *duration* of early morning stiffness.

4. Any associated symptoms.

The pattern of joint symptoms

The difference between the pattern of different rheumatic diseases is often an excellent guide to the diagnosis from the history alone:

(a) Soft tissue rheumatism (also called peri-arthritis or non-articular rheumatism) commonly affects tendons and bursae (Table 1).

(b) Primary OA affects a distinct pattern of joints (Table 2, Figure 3).

(c) Although a monoarthritis is not uncommon in some patients with inflammatory arthritis (particularly gout, pseudo-gout, reactive arthritis, psoriatic arthritis and some patients with RA), a history of a polyarthritis should always raise the possibility of inflammatory arthritis.

Always consider and exclude septic arthritis as a cause of monoarthritis.

Pain localized to one or two joints is more commonly due to either soft tissue rheumatism or OA. For example, a painful elbow joint is more likely to be due to an epicondylitis, as

Common sites of soft tissue rheumatism

The hand or wrist (tenosynovitis, e.g. De Quervain's tenosynovitis)

The elbow (epicondylitis – tennis elbow, golfer's elbow, olecranon bursitis)

The shoulder (rotator cuff tendonitis, subacromial bursitis, capsulitis)

The "hip" (trochanteric bursitis)

The knee (pre-patella bursitis)
The heel (Achilles tendonitis, plantar fasciitis)

Table 1. Common sites of soft tissue rheumatism.

Joints affected with primary OA

The distal interphalangeal joints (Heberden's nodes)

The proximal interphalangeal joints (Bouchard's nodes)

The carpo-metacarpal joints of the thumbs

The cervical spine (pain often referred to the scapula or shoulder)

The lumbar spine (pain often referred to the gluteal region or "hip")

The hip joints (pain is antero-medial)

The knee joints

The first metatarso-phalangeal joints

Table 2. Joints affected with primary OA.

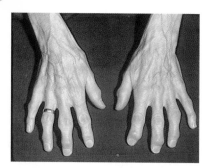

Figure 3. Nodal OA: Heberden's and Bouchard's nodes.

primary OA does not affect the elbow and it would be uncommon for an inflammatory arthritis only to affect the elbow.

Although those who complain of pain in several joints may also have OA, remember the joints that are *not* usually affected by OA (wrist, elbow, shoulder, ankle), as this would raise the possibility of other diagnoses. The inflammatory joint diseases should always be considered in a patient with polyarticular symptoms, but fibromyalgia should also be part of the differential diagnosis. A careful history of associated features is essential (described below).

Consider whether pain is referred. Pain is nearly always referred distally not proximally. It is common for patients to complain of shoulder pain or pain in the arms when referred from the cervical spine (Figure 4), and to complain of pain in the "hip" when the pain is referred from the lumbar spine. Pain arising from the hip joint is usually felt in the groin or radiates into the upper inner thigh and occasionally to the knee.

Joint swelling

Bony swelling occurs in OA and joint effusions may develop, but a clear history of joint swelling should always raise the possibility of inflammatory arthritis. Ensure the patient has not described the normal fluctuation in size of the digits from changes in ambient temperature.

The presence of synovial swelling detected on clinical examination is of considerable diagnostic importance (Figure 5).

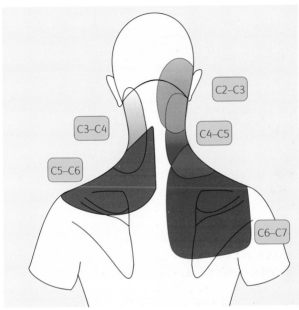

Figure 4. Distribution of pain referred from the cervical spine. Reproduced with permission from Linkaker CH *et al. Ballieres Clin Rheumatol* 1999; **13**: 197–215

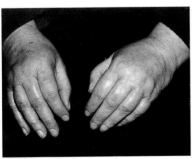

Figure 5. Synovial swelling in the metacarpo-phalangeal joints.

Early morning stiffness

Morning stiffness is a symptom of stiffness present on waking that eases with time. If the patient cannot describe any reduction in stiffness as the day progresses, the stiffness should not be considered to be "morning stiffness" (it is only in patients with the most severe inflammatory disease that morning stiffness lasts for the whole day). Morning stiffness of short duration is common in many people without arthritis and is certainly common in OA. *Prolonged* early morning stiffness is a symptom of inflammation and the duration tends to be correlated with the degree of inflammation. The severity or intensity of the stiffness does not have any diagnostic significance, nor does morning stiffness of short duration, whereas morning stiffness lasting for more than an hour is suggestive of inflammatory disease. However, there may be little morning stiffness if the inflammatory arthritis is either mild or in remission, and prolonged morning stiffness is a feature of some patients with fibromyalgia.

Ask the patient, "Do you feel stiff first thing in the morning?" and then ask "How long does it take to loosen up – less than 10 minutes, half an hour, an hour, two hours?" Record the duration of morning stiffness in minutes.

Associated features

In addition to a routine symptoms enquiry, any other history of the following should be documented.

Prodromal symptoms

Enquire about any prodromal symptoms, for example a recent history of a *viral illness*, *rash*, *conjunctivitis*, or a recent history of *diarrhoea or dysuria* that may have triggered a reactive arthritis.

Eye disease

Keratoconjunctivitis sicca is associated with most of the connective tissue diseases and may indicate either primary or secondary Sjögren's syndrome. A history of *iritis* (anterior uveitis; Figure 6) is a strong indication of a sero-negative spondylo-arthritis.

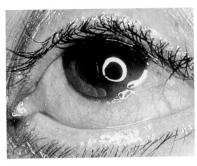

Figure 6. Acute iritis (anterior uveitis).

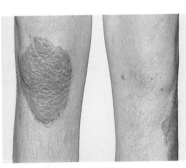

Figure 7. Psoriasis.

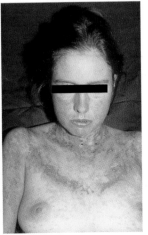

Figure 8. Butterfly rash and severe photosensitive rash from systemic lupus erythematosus (SLE).

Skin rash

A history of *psoriasis* (Figure 7) would clearly be relevant. A history of *photosensitivity* or alopecia, particularly in a young woman with joint pain, should raise the possibility of systemic lupus erythematosus (SLE) (Figure 8).

Ask the patient, "Have you ever had psoriasis" (patients may not recall a minor episode of psoriasis in the past if they are only asked whether they suffer from skin rashes).

Raynaud's phenomenon

Raynaud's phenomenon is common in young women without joint disease, but does raise the possibility of an auto-immune disease.

Pleuritic pain

SLE should be considered if there is a previous history of *pleurisy* or *pericarditis*, particularly in young women.

Inflammatory bowel disease

Enteropathic arthritis is a common feature of *inflammatory bowel disease*. Although the diagnosis usually predates the onset of joint disease, arthritis may occasionally develop in patients prior to a diagnosis of either Crohn's disease or ulcerative colitis, and any history of abdominal pain or diarrhoea in a patient with joint pain should be determined.

Systemic symptoms

Weight loss or other systemic symptoms, including *anorexia* or *night sweats*, are important symptoms and raise the possibility of serious illness. Always consider whether the rheumatic symptoms may be a manifestation of malignancy, or other serious diseases such as polyarteritis nodosa.

Obstetric history

A past history of *recurrent spontaneous abortion* should raise the possibility of anti-phospholipid syndrome.[5]

Family history

A family history of OA or RA is often unhelpful, unless there is a particularly strong history in several close family members. The familial association of these conditions is relatively weak, but a family history of psoriasis, iritis, inflammatory bowel disease or ankylosing spondylitis is often more relevant in view of the known genetic link (HLA-B27) between these diseases.[6]

Clinical examination

General examination

Observation of the patient walking into the consulting room is important. Is there evidence of stiffness in movement, or a limp? Does the patient have any evidence of weight loss or pallor suggestive of serious illness? Are there any skin rashes? If an inflammatory arthritis is suspected, look particularly for psoriasis in the nails, scalp and extensor surfaces of the elbows and knees. Bony swelling may indicate Paget's disease (Figure 9).

Examination of the joints

It is advisable to examine all the joints, even when the symptoms are localized, as there may be signs in other joints that are not symptomatic. Always compare the same joint on each side of the body. It only takes a few minutes to examine all joints for the following:

1. Erythema.
2. Range of movement.
3. Deformity.
4. Soft tissue swelling.
5. Joint effusions.
6. Bony swelling.
7. Crepitus.
8. Tenderness.
9. Muscle wasting or weakness.
10. Nerve root entrapment.

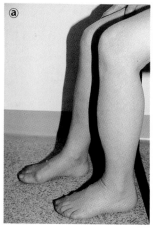 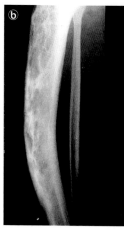

Figure 9. (A) Paget's disease of the left tibia. (B) X-ray of Paget's disease in the tibia.

Erythema is a feature of acute rather than chronic inflammation and raises the possibility of sepsis, metabolic arthritis or reactive arthritis.

Hands

- Always start with an examination of the hands (over 25% of joints in the body are in the hands and wrists). Evaluate the range of movement by asking the patient to make a fist; then ask the patient to put both hands together as in prayer with the wrists fully extended, then with the dorsal aspects of the hands opposed and the wrists fully flexed.
- Is there any subluxation or other deformity of any joints?
- Look for synovial swelling, particularly in a rheumatoid distribution – proximal interphalangeal (PIP) joints, metacarpo-phalangeal (MCP) joints and wrists (Figure 10).
- Is there any bony swelling and/or tenderness in the carpo-metacarpal (CMC) joint of the thumb, or bony swelling in the distal interphalangeal (DIP) joints and PIPs suggestive of OA?
- Is there any swelling or tenderness in the extensor tendons, particularly over the dorsum of the wrist, or the

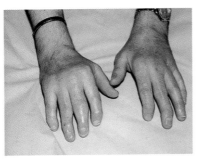

Figure 10.
Rheumatoid type
psoriatic arthritis –
note psoriasis of the
nails.

flexor tendons, particularly in the palm of the hand?
If there is localized pain, is there pain in any tendon on
resisted flexion or extension of the thumb, fingers or
wrists, or crepitus in the tendons on passive movement?
- Is there wasting of the thenar eminence, or in the other
small muscles of the hands?

Elbows
- Ask the patient to fully flex then fully extend the elbows.
- Examine the skin over the extensor surface of the elbow
for psoriasis.
- Is there swelling or tenderness of the olecranon bursa
or any nodules or gouty tophi in the bursa (Figure 11)?
- Palpate the groove between the olecranon and lateral
epicondyle for any synovial swelling and tenderness
indicative of an inflammatory arthritis.
- Is there tenderness over the medial or lateral epicondyle
suggesting tennis or golfer's elbow?

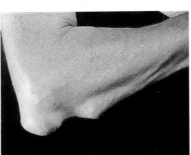

Figure 11.
Rheumatoid nodules.

Shoulders

- The shoulder joint has the greatest range of movement of any joint. Evaluate movement in flexion, extension, abduction, adduction, internal and external rotation. Ask the patient to raise the arms first forwards, then backwards, sideways in abduction, then put the hand behind the back as far as possible to assess internal rotation.
- Is there swelling or tenderness? Tenderness under the lateral acromion is suggestive of a rotator cuff lesion.
- Passively raising the arm in an arc whilst holding the acromion to prevent shrugging is painful if there is subacromial impingement from a rotator cuff lesion.
- Resisted abduction and resisted external rotation evaluate the supraspinatus and infraspinatus tendons separately. If there is weakness without pain, consider whether there may be either a rotator cuff tear or a neurological cause such as a radiculopathy.
- Pain with resisted flexion of the elbow (with the palm facing upwards) is indicative of biceps tendinitis.
- Look at the shoulder from behind. Is there any muscle wasting around the shoulder or scapula suggestive of a radiculopathy?

Neck

- Ask the patient to extend the neck as far as possible, then put the chin on the chest, then each ear in turn on the shoulder. Take into account that the range of normal movement of the cervical spine gradually reduces with age.
- Is there any tenderness located to one vertebra or muscle?
- Is there tenderness at the point of muscle insertion in the occiput?
- Is there any muscle spasm, weakness or wasting?

Lumbar spine

- Examine the spine with the patient standing. Is there any asymmetry from a scoliosis? A physiological scoliosis will correct on flexion.

- Is there any limitation of movement in flexion, extension, rotation and lateral flexion? The (modified) Schober's test (Figure 12) is a useful guide – with the patient standing upright, mark two points with a pen 15 cm apart, approximately 10 cm above and 5 cm below the dimples of Venus. Ask the patient to bend forward as far as possible to try and touch the toes, then measure the distance between the points. Normal flexion is an increase of at least 5 cm.
- Gently thump the spine and sacro-iliac joints. A localized area of bone pain and tenderness may indicate serious pathology.
- With the patient prone evaluate the femoral stretch test – put your left hand under the knee and extend the hip, then with your right hand flex the knee as far as possible. Pain and muscle spasm indicate nerve root entrapment at L3 or L4.
- With the patient supine and with the opposite knee flexed, lift each leg in turn as far as possible with the knee extended then dorsiflex the ankle. Pain and muscle spasm will reduce the degree of straight leg raising if there is significant nerve root entrapment at L5 or S1.

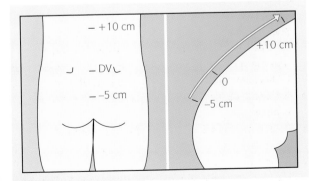

Figure 12. Modified Schober's test. DV, dimples of Venus. Reproduced with kind permission of the Arthritis Research Campaign (www.arc.org.uk).

- Assess the power of the extensors of the great toe – weakness may indicate a lesion at L5.
- Weakness of ankle dorsiflexion may indicate a lesion at L4 or L5.
- Test the tendon reflexes. A depressed knee jerk indicates a lesion at L3/L4 and a depressed ankle jerk at S1.

Hips

- Examine the hips with the patient in a supine position. The most important signs are reduced range of movement and pain on movement.
- Is there any muscle wasting of the quadriceps or buttocks?
- Is there flexion beyond 90°?
- With the hip flexed, assess passive internal and external rotation (Figure 13) – ask the patient to allow the leg to fall inwards and outwards as far as possible.
- Place one hand on the contralateral iliac crest (to assess any pelvic rotation), then take the weight of the leg and assess the degree of (passive) abduction of the hip.
- Palpate over the greater trochanter – tenderness is indicative of a bursitis.

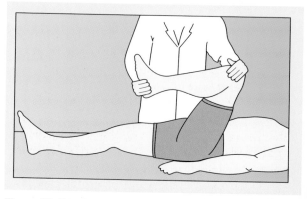

Figure 13. Examination of the hip joint – flexion, internal and external rotation. Reproduced with kind permission of the Arthritis Research Campaign (www.arc.org.uk).

Knees

- Evaluate the range of flexion and extension while palpating for crepitus. Flexion deformity of the knee is disabling and unless long-standing is an indication for urgent treatment.
- Is there any wasting of the quadriceps muscles?
- Look for any deformity. Valgus deformity is less common than varus deformity in OA and may indicate an inflammatory arthritis (Figure 14).

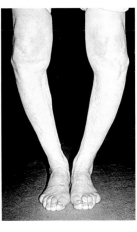

Figure 14. Varus deformity from OA of the knees.

- Is there any swelling? Bursal swellings are a common and often incidental finding unless they are tender.
- A small effusion may be detected at the medial side of the patella when the normal concave contour of the knee is lost. Attempt to "milk" the fluid from this area – observing the fluid return is confirmatory evidence of an effusion. A positive patella tap sign (elicited by feeling a small tap when sharply depressing the patella; Figure 15) may not be present when there is either a very small or a very large effusion. Synovial swelling is usually diffuse and may be difficult to differentiate from an effusion, although it should be possible to demonstrate that an effusion is fluctuant.

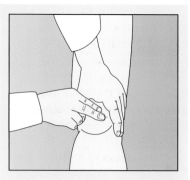

Figure 15. Patella tap sign. Reproduced with kind permission of the Arthritis Research Campaign (www.arc.org.uk).

- Palpate the popliteal fossa. A popliteal (Baker's) cyst may be visible with the patient standing and is usually felt on the medial side of the fossa.
- Evaluate the lateral movement of the patella. Marked laxity may indicate a problem with tracking of the patella.
- Is there tenderness? With the knee flexed, a localized tender area either medially or laterally just below the patella may indicate a meniscal lesion.
- Evaluate any lateral instability – with the knee extended, fix the leg above the knee with your left hand and with your right hand hold the leg above the ankle and attempt to rock the lower leg sideways.
- Examine the cruciate ligaments with the anterior draw test – with the knee flexed at 90°, hold the lower leg with both hands and gently pull forwards.

Ankles and feet
- Look at both flexion/extension from the ankle joint and eversion/inversion from the sub-talar joint.
- Examine the Achilles tendon for tenderness or swelling.
- Look for synovial swelling anteriorly and around the malleoli.
- Look at the alignment of the ankle with the patient standing. It is often easier to see any deformity by examining the ankle from behind the patient.

- With the patient still standing, examine the arch of the foot for any pes planus (Figure 16).
- Is there any bony swelling, especially of the first metatarso-phalangeal (MTP) joint, indicative of OA or valgus deformity of the hallux causing a bunion?
- Is there any upward subluxation of the toes or deviation?
- Synovial swelling in the MTP joints may be suggested by separation of the toes (daylight sign), but is often not obvious.
- Is there any tenderness of the forefoot or the MTP joints – squeezing the foot firmly across the metatarsals will be painful if there is synovitis (Figure 17).

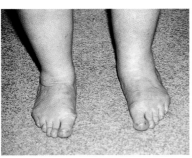

Figure 16. Valgus deformity of the ankles with pes planus and hallux rigidus.

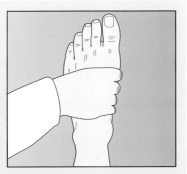

Figure 17. Squeeze the metatarsals to detect synovitis. Reproduced with kind permission of the Arthritis Research Campaign (www.arc.org.uk).

Investigations

General principles

Investigations need to be appropriate to the clinical presentation, as there is little value in a battery of screening investigations. They should be undertaken to address a specific question, and the results used to support or refute a clinical diagnosis. For example, there is no point in undertaking a rheumatoid factor in a patient presenting with back pain: RA does not present with back pain and a number of patients will have a false-positive result, which may lead to unnecessary anxiety and further investigations. Conversely, many patients with recent onset of RA may have completely normal investigations. X-rays may also confuse rather than enlighten. There is little value in taking an X-ray of the cervical spine in an elderly patient with neck and shoulder pain to determine if there is cervical spondylosis: radiographic changes of spondylosis are universal in elderly people and correlate poorly with symptoms.[7]

Some simple investigations are appropriate in most patients. A test of the acute phase response is advisable in nearly all patients. If it is unexpectedly elevated, it should raise the possibility of inflammatory arthritis. Most patients should also have a blood count. The presence of anaemia may either be an indication of systemic or inflammatory disease, but may also develop secondary to upper gastrointestinal blood loss from anti-inflammatory drugs.

Immunological investigations should be undertaken if there are clinical features of inflammatory arthritis. However, a number of auto-antibodies may occur in low titre in people without arthritis, and a "false-positive" result is often misleading unless it is in taken in context with the clinical presentation.[8]

If the symptoms and signs are diagnostic of OA, then investigations other than a blood count and ESR may be unnecessary and potentially misleading.

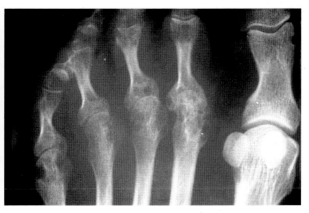

Figure 18. Erosions and subluxation of the MTP joints from RA.

X-ray appearances of OA are common and age related. They should therefore be undertaken either to assess the severity of OA or to look for erosions in patients who may have an inflammatory arthritis (Figure 18).

Remember that, in early disease, the majority of patients with RA have normal X-rays and 50% have a negative rheumatoid factor. In mild disease, the acute phase investigations may also be normal. The diagnosis is made on clinical criteria.

Other investigations should be considered if there is a suspicion of serious illness, although it is inappropriate to be specific. Investigations may include a blood count, ESR and CRP, serum calcium and alkaline phosphatase, serum and urinary electrophoresis to exclude myeloma, and a prostate-specific antigen in men. A chest X-ray looking for primary or secondary tumour, X-rays of the site of pain and an isotope bone scan may all be indicated. The clinical features should dictate the need for other investigations.

General Principles of Management

Principles of treatment

Treatment should always be considered as both general and specific. General measures of treatment apply to any patient with rheumatic symptoms. Specific treatment is discussed in the relevant sections.

General measures

This advice is applicable to all patients with rheumatic symptoms, and is considered in three areas (Figure 19):

(a)   joint protection;
(b)   exercises;
(c)   simple pain relief.

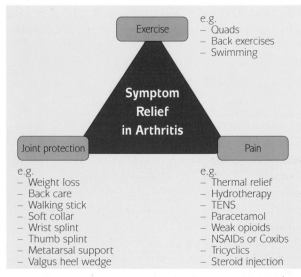

Figure 19. Symptom relief in arthritis.

Joint protection
Weight loss
Obesity is often associated with joint pain, and losing weight is important both for pain relief and to reduce the progression of OA in weight-bearing joints. Losing weight in patients who are inactive because of arthritis is particularly difficult, but should be regularly encouraged because of the delay in progression of disease in those able to achieve significant weight loss.[9]

Posture and activities
Advice should be given in order to restrict painful joints from being overused. This may mean giving advice to patients with neck or shoulder pain or back pain to avoid simple everyday activities such as heavy housework, e.g. cleaning windows, hanging curtains, and to avoid carrying heavy shopping or digging the garden. Enquire about posture and potential stress on the joints for those at work. Is it possible to advise a simple modification to posture at work that may reduce stress on painful joints? Participation in sports may be beneficial, but activities that directly cause pain should be avoided. Discuss a change in sport or exercise – for example, swimming may be better than jogging for those with pain in the back or lower limbs. Give specific advice when appropriate.

Do not assume that because the advice seems obvious that it is not worth giving.

Aids and appliances
Give advice about simple aids and appliances that will either protect joint position or reduce joint strain, e.g.:
* *Walking stick*: should be recommended for arthritis in the hip or knee of moderate severity, carried in the contralateral hand to the worst symptoms. The stick should be long enough so that the elbow is slightly flexed. Those who initially refuse to consider a walking stick may be encouraged to use a stout umbrella.

- *Foam collar*: sleeping in a *narrow* soft collar (Figure 20) – approximately 2.5 inches (6.5 cm) in diameter – protects against an exacerbation of symptoms from abnormal posture and should be advised at the onset of symptoms.[10] Deeper collars may exacerbate symptoms and are not recommended for sleep. (Those intolerant to a collar may try either a sculpted pillow or a "butterfly" pillow – tie a ribbon tightly round the centre of a soft pillow.)

- *Thumb splint* (Figure 21): should be advised for all those with pain in the CMC joint of the thumb from OA and De Quervain's tenosynovitis.
  The splint should be worn for lifting or any manual work. The choice between an elasticated or neoprene splint is dictated by comfort.

- *Wrist splint* (Figure 22): indicated for carpal tunnel syndrome, tenosynovitis of the wrist and inflammatory arthritis of the wrist.

- *Tennis elbow splint*: these are occasionally helpful for tennis or golfer's elbow by restricting pronation and supination.

- *Lumbar support*: it is preferable to avoid strong supports and corsets for the majority of those with back pain because of the possibility of increasing muscle weakness. Lightweight supports may be recommended to be used at times of greatest activity, e.g. gardening, as the support will remind the patient to avoid stooping.

- *Valgus heel wedge*: indicated for pain in the foot and ankle associated with a valgus deformity in the ankle.

- *Heel pad*: sorbothane or other shock-absorbing rubber heel pads (Figure 23) are indicated for heel pain, ankle pain and Achilles tendinitis.

- *Metatarsal pads*: these may be applied to an insole or strapped to the forefoot and reduce symptoms from forefoot pain particularly when there is metatarsal tenderness.

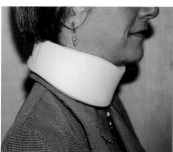

Figure 20. Narrow soft foam collar.

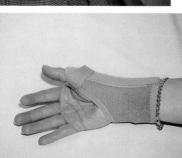

Figure 21. Thumb splint.

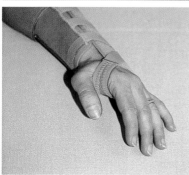

Figure 22. Wrist splint.

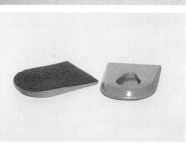

Figure 23. Sorbothane heel pads.

Exercises

Muscle wasting results from the reduction in muscle tone in muscle groups that act upon any painful or swollen joint. Active exercises are an essential part of the management of all patients with arthritis, and should be undertaken to maintain and improve muscle strength. This leads to a reduction in both disability and pain.[11,12] In addition, passive exercises are important for those with inflammatory arthritis in order to maintain a full range of movement in an inflamed joint. Swimming should be encouraged in most patients with arthritis, although it may exacerbate symptoms in some patients with neck pain.

Physical methods of pain relief
Thermal treatment

Application of heat or cold is often effective in offering short-lived pain relief and all patients should be given advice on how to do this at home. It is individual preference whether to use a hot water bottle, a heat pack, hot wax or a heat lamp. Patients should be advised to apply heat to the painful muscles or joints, especially before undertaking exercises. Although it is unlikely that any persistent benefit will be achieved, hot packs can be used frequently for pain relief. Cold packs may be more effective in some patients, and should be recommended in patients with a poor response to heat or if there is an acutely painful and swollen joint. Cold packs are also helpful after acute injury. Always reassure the patient that the application of hot or cold packs will not aggravate or cause deterioration in joint disease, but to take care to avoid a skin burn.

Hydrotherapy

Similar advice should be given about the value of a hot bath or shower. This is often effective in reducing pain and stiffness in the muscles and joints. A showerhead can be directed to a local area of pain and help to relieve symptoms. Immersing the hands in hot water can be undertaken frequently during the day in patients with pain in the small joints of the hands.

Wearing rubber gloves allows a higher water temperature to be tolerated, often with better relief of symptoms.

Trans-cutaneous electrical stimulation (TENS)

A TENS machine applies a small electrical current to the skin over an area of pain and helps to relieve pain during the period it is used. It is a counter irritant and may stimulate the release of endorphins in some patients. Although it is helpful in some patients, it should be recommended initially only on a trial basis. Some patients find it invaluable; others find it worthless.

Simple drug therapy

Paracetamol (acetaminophen) up to 1 g q.i.d. should be recommended as an adjunct to the advice on joint protection, exercises and physical methods of pain relief. If ineffective, a paracetamol–weak opioid preparation may be prescribed with or without a therapeutic trial of a non-steroidal anti-inflammatory drug (NSAID) or cyclo-oxygenase-2 inhibitor (coxib). Consider an intra-articular or intralesional steroid injection for localized pain. Low dose tricyclic antidepressant should also be considered for chronic pain. Drug treatment is discussed in more detail on pp 37–50.

When to refer to a rheumatologist

Referral to a rheumatologist should be considered in three different circumstances:

1. If there is uncertainty in the diagnosis.
2. Any patient who fails to have a good response to treatment.
3. All patients with a diagnosis of inflammatory joint disease (with the exception of uncomplicated gout and polymyalgia rheumatica).

A confident diagnosis is necessary in order to institute an appropriate regime of treatment and to offer advice on prognosis. If a diagnosis of an inflammatory joint disease is considered, it is essential to refer to a rheumatologist for an opinion and management. The purpose of this visit would be to confirm the diagnosis and to indicate whether specific drug treatment is required which may affect the prognosis.

Patients who fail to respond to treatment may benefit from a review by a rheumatologist in order to confirm the diagnosis and make any further recommendations that may be appropriate. Patients may also benefit from being referred to other hospital services such as physiotherapy and occupational therapy or for surgical appliances.

When to refer to an orthopaedic surgeon

The majority of patients with arthritis do not require surgical treatment. Consider a surgical referral in those with any instability of the joints or other potential mechanical abnormality and those with pain unresponsive to other treatment, particularly when associated with radiological appearances of severe arthritis.

The following is a general guide:

- *Carpal tunnel syndrome* – failure to respond to conservative treatment, including wrist splints and occasional glucocorticoid injection.
- *Shoulder pain* – failure to respond to steroid injections plus either severe pain or weakness.
- *Neck pain* – severe pain radiating down the arm unresponsive to drug therapy and a soft collar during the night, or the development of a neurological deficit.
- *Back pain* – severe pain radiating down the leg with signs of nerve root entrapment (reduced straight leg raising, positive femoral stretch test, asymmetrical tendon reflexes). Urgent referral if there is sphincter disturbance suggestive of cauda equina syndrome.
- *Hip pain* – severe changes of OA on X-ray plus significant disability and severe pain in a typical distribution occurring at rest (including nocturnal pain), despite full medical treatment.
- *Knee pain* – moderate to severe changes of OA on X-ray plus significant disability and pain, usually worse with walking, despite full medical treatment.
- *Ankle and foot pain* – severe pain despite full modification of the footwear and full medical treatment.

Drug Treatment

Simple analgesia

Paracetamol (acetaminophen) is a safe and effective compound, and is commonly considered as the analgesic of first choice. However, if there is severe pain in the context of inflammation then a NSAID or a coxib should be considered first. Adverse events from paracetamol are rare but can be serious. Interactions with other compounds are rare. Care must be taken in advising the patient to be careful about the use of combinations of over the counter products that might expose them to unexpectedly higher acetaminophen doses. Doses up to 1 g q.i.d. should be recommended before considering other analgesics. Paracetamol in combination with opioid derivatives should be recommended when there is inadequate pain relief to paracetamol alone. Available preparations include combinations with codeine (co-codamol), dextropropoxyphene (co-proxamol) and dihydrocodeine (co-dydramol). In some patients, it may be preferable to prescribe the opioid separately rather than in a fixed combination with paracetamol. However, many patients will take different combinations of paracetamol or paracetamol/opioid compounds depending on daily symptoms. There is considerable variation in response to treatment, and some patients have significant side-effects from the opioids, including drowsiness and constipation. Other opioids such as tramadol may be better tolerated and may be prescribed alone or in addition to paracetamol, although the dose should be slowly increased to minimize the potential for toxic effects.

Many patients will have adequate control of their symptoms with this advice. For those with persistent symptoms, providing there has been some response, the paracetamol or paracetamol/opioid combination may be continued as required in addition to anti-inflammatories and other treatment.

NSAIDs

Non-steroidal anti-inflammatory drugs (NSAIDs) have weak analgesic effects in addition to their anti-inflammatory properties. They are particularly helpful at relieving stiffness, perhaps predictably as this is a symptom of inflammation. The analgesic effect is often more pronounced in patients with an inflammatory component to their arthritis, but in crossover studies (Figure 24) NSAIDs are also preferred to paracetamol in more than 50% of patients with OA.[13,14] NSAIDs should always be prescribed as a therapeutic trial. Patients should be informed that these drugs do not have any protective or long-term benefits and should only be continued if the symptomatic benefit is greater than that from simple analgesia.

NSAIDs should be used with caution in patients with renal disease, cardiac failure and obstructive airways disease. However, the major side-effects are related to the upper gastrointestinal (GI) tract. Dyspepsia is common but is a poor indication of gastric damage, as most gastric ulcers are silent.[15,16] Approximately 15–20% of patients taking NSAIDs will have an ulcer at any one point in time; gastric ulcers are twice as common as duodenal ulcers. Those at greatest risk of developing an ulcer and ulcer complications are the elderly and frail, especially those with co-morbid diseases and disability, or those with a previous history of ulceration or ulcer complications.[17–19] The mortality from the GI complications of NSAIDs is a major public health problem (Figure 25).[20] Elderly patients should not be prescribed NSAIDs unless they have failed other therapy (including coxibs) and should *never* be prescribed in the elderly without co-prescription of cytoprotective drugs. Misoprostol reduces the risk of ulceration and ulcer complications by approximately 50%.[21,22] Fixed combination preparations of misoprostol with diclofenac are as effective in prophylaxis of ulcers as co-prescription, but may be preferred in the elderly not only for ease of administration but in order to improve compliance.[23]

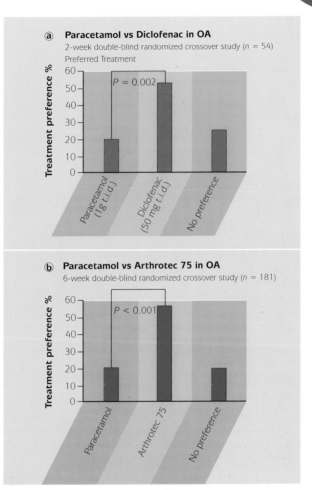

Figure 24. Treatment preference of patients in crossover studies: paracetamol vs NSAIDs. Part A reproduced by permission of Oxford University Press from Pickavance L, Griffiths G, McKenna F. *Br J Rheumatol* 1995; **34**(Supply 1): 37.[13] Part B used by permission of Wiley-Liss, Inc. a subsidary of John Wiley & Sons, Inc. from Pincus T, Koch GG, Sokka T *et al. Arth Rheum* 2000; **44**: 1587–1598.[14]

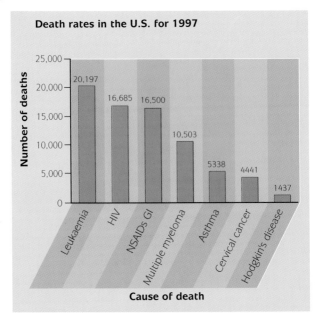

Figure 25. Mortality rates from NSAID-induced gastrointestinal damage. Reproduced with permission from National Center for Health Statistics, 1998.

H$_2$ antagonists are not effective in preventing gastric ulceration from NSAIDs[24,25] except in high dose.[26] Proton pump inhibitors appear to have similar benefits to misoprostol and are significantly more effective than H$_2$ antagonists in preventing damage.[27,28] However, co-prescription of cyto-protective drugs will only reduce and not eliminate the risk.

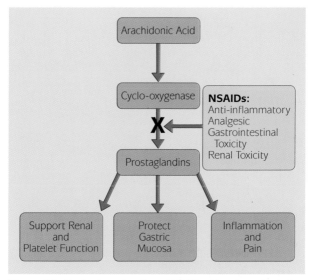

Figure 26. Mechanism of action of NSAIDs: Vane hypothesis.

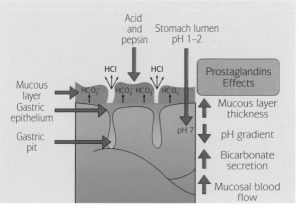

Figure 27. Normal gastric protective mechanisms. Adapted from references 31 and 32.

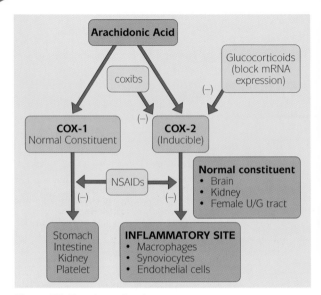

Figure 28. Functions of cyclo-oxygenase enzymes.

COX-2 inhibitors (coxibs)

The hypothesis that the mode of action of NSAIDs was a result of the inhibition of the cyclo-oxygenase enzyme was proposed more than three decades ago (Figure 26).[29] Inhibition of the enzyme leads to a reduction in pro-inflammatory prostaglandins, but also leads to a reduction in prostaglandins involved in maintaining mucosal integrity in the stomach and duodenum,[31, 32] and in platelet function and renal homeostasis (Figure 27).

In the late 1980s it was established that there were at least two different cyclo-oxygenase enzymes, subsequently termed COX-1 and COX-2.[30] COX-1 is a constitutive enzyme largely responsible for normal body homeostasis, whereas COX-2 is predominantly induced as part of the inflammatory process. COX-2 also has some constitutive functions but is not found in platelets or normal GI mucosa (Figure 28).

A number of compounds have now been developed which selectively inhibit COX-2 while sparing COX-1 in therapeutic

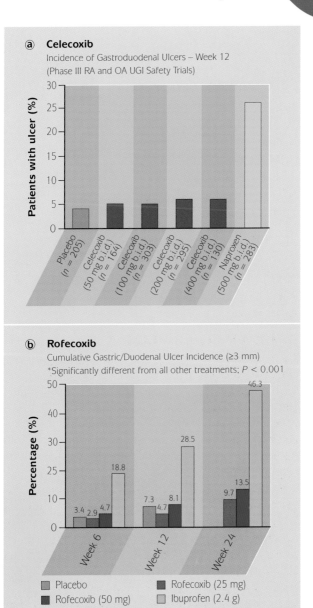

Figure 29. Incidence of ulcers using coxibs.

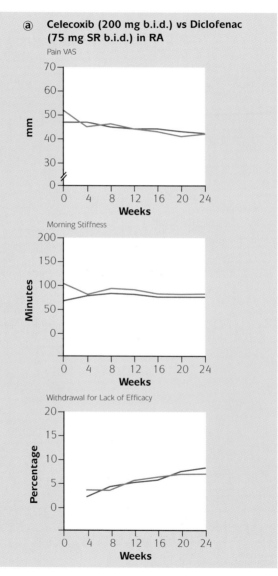

Figure 30. Efficacy of celecoxib vs diclofenac in the treatment of arthritis. VAS, visual analogue scale. Parts A and B reproduced with permission from Elsevier Science (The Lancet 1999; **354**:

ⓑ **Celecoxib (200 mg b.i.d.) vs Diclofenac (75 mg SR b.i.d.) in RA (cont.)**

No. of Tender/Painful Joints

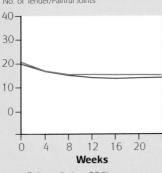

— Celecoxib (n=326)
— Diclofenac (n=329)

ⓒ **Celecoxib (100 mg b.i.d.) vs Diclofenac (50 mg t.i.d.) in OA**

Patient's Assessment of Pain

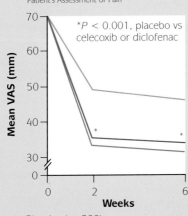

— Placebo (n=200)
— Celecoxib (100 mg b.i.d; n=199)
— Diclofenac (50 mg t.i.d; n=199)

2106)[35]. Part C used data from McKenna F, Borenstein D, Wendt H, Wallemark C, Lefkowith J, Geis GS. *Scand J Rheum* 2001; **30**: 11–18.[36]

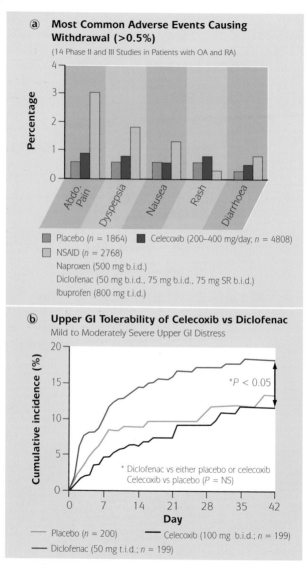

Figure 31. Adverse events and GI tolerability of celecoxib vs NSAIDs. Reproduced with permission from McKenna F, Arguelles L, Burke T, Lefkowith J, Geis GS. *Clin Exp Rheumatol* 2002; **20**: 35–43.[37]

doses. These drugs have been given the generic name of coxibs and have been found to have similar efficacy to the NSAIDs, but with a placebo incidence of endoscopic damage on the upper GI tract (Figure 29).[33, 34]

Celecoxib was the first drug in this new class to be developed and marketed. Extensive studies have found that celecoxib has the same efficacy as a range of standard NSAIDs in the treatment of both RA and OA (Figure 30).[35, 36]

In addition to a placebo incidence of gastric and duodenal ulceration, it has almost a placebo incidence of dyspepsia (Figure 31).[37]

Studies with other coxibs have found similar efficacy and reduction in serious GI toxicity.[38, 39] Rofecoxib, valdecoxib and etoricoxib have been licensed in many countries, and are as effective as other comparator NSAIDs, although there may be some minor differences in tolerability. Long-term outcome studies have found a significant reduction in serious complications, including GI haemorrhage and perforation.[40, 41] The adverse effects on the kidney also appear to be reduced, although in view of the physiological role of COX-2 in the kidney,[42] coxibs should be used with caution in patients with renal impairment and cardiac failure.

NICE criteria of patients at risk from NSAIDs

1. Age > 65 years
2. Previous history of gastroduodenal ulcer, perforation, or GI haemorrhage
3. Concomitant use of medications that increase the likelihood of GI adverse events (e.g. steroids and anticoagulants)
4. Presence of serious co-morbidity, such as cardiovascular disease, renal or hepatic impairment, diabetes and hypertension
5. Requirement for the prolonged use of maximum recommended doses of standard NSAIDs

Table 3. NICE criteria of patients at risk from NSAIDs.

The long-term outcome study with rofecoxib also raised concerns about a possible increase in myocardial infarction (MI) from coxibs. However, this has not been seen in the long-term studies with celecoxib, and it is likely that the observations with rofecoxib could be explained by one of three observations: that it was a chance finding, or from a degree of cardio-protection from the anti-platelet effects of naproxen,[43] the comparator NSAID or it could have been caused by rofecoxib. There has been no prospectively collected data to suggest that naproxen will decrease the incidence of MI and it should not be used to provide cardioprotection.

The availability of safer and effective therapy has raised further questions about the safety of NSAIDs. It is likely that most NSAIDs will become redundant once a number of coxibs are available on generic prescription. The indications to prescribe a coxib in preference to an NSAID have been defined in the UK by the National Institute for Clinical Excellence (NICE) (Table 3).

Corticosteroids

Steroids can be administered as regular oral doses, as pulse oral, intravenous or intramuscular doses, or by intra-articular injection. Side-effects are related to the total dose (Table 4).

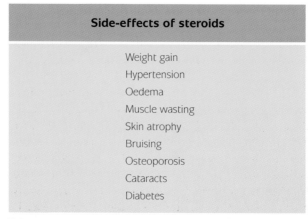

Side-effects of steroids
Weight gain
Hypertension
Oedema
Muscle wasting
Skin atrophy
Bruising
Osteoporosis
Cataracts
Diabetes

Table 4. Side-effects of steroids.

Pulse steroids are used in patients with inflammatory arthritis in inducing a short improvement in disease activity and are recommended when initiating or changing disease-modifying anti-rheumatoid drugs.[44–46] The choice of therapy varies depending on the experience of the prescribing rheumatologist. There are advantages of intramuscular steroids (80 mg triamcinolone acetonide or 80–120 mg methylprednisolone), as there is no risk of the treatment being continued by the patient and may be more effective than equivalent oral doses. High dose pulse intravenous methylprednisolone may be administered in resistant cases when other drug treatment has failed and is often used in conjunction with intravenous cyclophosphamide for the treatment of vasculitis.[47]

It is important to administer triamcinolone as a deep intramuscular injection because of the risk of subcutaneous fat atrophy resulting in a disfiguring dimple or scar.

Intra-articular steroids should be considered for the treatment of synovitis of a small number of joints or for treatment of the most active joints in conjunction with other treatment. Intra-articular steroids are also effective in some patients with OA, particularly when there are signs of inflammation such as a joint effusion. Intralesional steroids are often effective for soft tissue lesions, including bursitis and tendinitis.

Triamcinolone is contraindicated for soft tissue injections because of the increased risk of a fat atrophy with this steroid.

Regular doses of oral steroids are avoided when possible because of the risk of side-effects. In addition, because the short-term benefits of higher doses are apparent, some patients may increase the dose above that prescribed despite the increased risk of side-effects. However, oral steroids are indicated for patients with inflammatory arthritis who have failed to respond to other treatment, for many elderly patients with RA and for the treatment of systemic complications. They are the only effective reatment for polymyalgia rheumatica, and form part of the treatment of many patients with other connective tissue diseases. The lowest effective dose should be prescribed and for chronic treatment should preferably not exceed 10 mg/day. Clinicans should not use oral glucocorticoids to treat OA, even when there is some evidence of inflammation.

Management of side-effects

- Screen patients for potential side-effects.
- Steroids stimulate the appetite, leading to weight gain. Advise all patients to be careful with diet.
- Check the blood pressure at each clinical review.
- Undertake regular urinalysis for glycosuria. Patients with latent diabetes mellitus may develop hyperglycaemia and often require treatment following the initiation of therapy. The blood glucose may return to normal after the steroids are withdrawn.
- Skin and muscle atrophy are a problem in those with prolonged high doses. Use the minimum effective dose and consider azathioprine or methotrexate to allow a reduction in steroid dose.
- Prophylaxis with daily supplements of calcium and vitamin D is recommended during prolonged steroid treatment.
- Measure the bone density in those at greatest risk and co-prescribe a biphosphonate if indicated.

Neuropsychiatric drugs

Tricyclic antidepressants

The tricyclic antidepressants (TCAs) are used widely in a variety of chronic pain states independent of any coexisting depression. Amitriptyline has been the most widely studied drug in chronic pain, although a number of others have also been used.[48] The sedating compounds are preferable as they help to reduce night waking from pain.

The mechanism of their analgesic action is uncertain. They may potentiate the endogenous opioid system.[49] It has also been suggested that their action as serotonin and norepinephrine reuptake inhibitors may be linked with their analgesic effects, although the selective serotonin re-uptake inhibitors (SSRIs) are not as effective as analgesics. Although TCAs may help to relieve the depressive symptoms associated with chronic pain, the effective doses are usually below those used for depression, and the lack of analgesia from more effective antidepressants such as SSRIs supports the presence of an independent analgesic effect.

Other than sedation, side-effects are relatively uncommon and are usually related to the anticholinergic effects on GI, cardiovascular and neurological systems, but are relatively contraindicated in patients with severe cardiac disease, particularly in those with conduction disturbances. The sedative side-effect is helpful in those with sleep disturbance from pain, and most patients will have a subjective improvement in their sleep pattern. There may be a hangover effect on waking in some patients, but this usually reduces over the first weeks of therapy. In order to reduce this effect, it is advisable to commence therapy on a low dose (e.g. 25 mg nocte) of amitryptiline or dothiepin, and increase gradually to a usual maintenance dose of 75 mg nocte. For those with a marked hangover effect, the dose could be taken earlier in the evening.

Anticonvulsants

Phenytoin, carbamazepine, sodium valproate, clonazepam, gabapentin and lamotrigine have all been used for chronic pain with variable results.[50] Their mechanisms of action are not fully understood. Phenytoin is known to have a membrane-stabilizing action that may be related to its analgesic effects, whereas sodium valproate and clonazepam may inhibit excitatory amines. Carbamazepine prevents repeated discharges in neurons and is most effective in trigeminal neuralgia. They tend to be used when all other treatment has failed. Adverse effects are common with most of the anticonvulsants, and initiation and monitoring of treatment are usually undertaken in secondary care.

Management of Soft Tissue Rheumatism

Fibromyalgia

This is a common cause of generalized rheumatic symptoms and occurs in up to 1% of the population.[4] It occurs predominantly in women aged 20–60 years and may be triggered by a viral illness or physical trauma. It can be considered as part of a spectrum of illness, including post-viral fatigue syndrome – often (incorrectly) termed "ME". Patients are usually low in mood, have a reduced exercise tolerance and frequently complain of malaise. Some patients have associated vascular or GI symptoms such as cold peripheries and abdominal cramps. There is often sleep disturbance and it has been postulated that this may be important as an aetiological factor from changes in delta wave sleep.[51]

The predominant symptoms are myalgia and arthralgia, often with prolonged morning stiffness. The majority of patients have pain in the neck and shoulder girdle, often with low back pain in addition to diffuse symptoms in the limbs. On examination, a characteristic finding is tenderness at "hyperalgesic points" in a number of sites in and around joints[52] (see Figure 32). Whether this is related to a reduction in pain threshold or due to a different pathological process is at present undetermined. The hyperalgesic points should be examined with the thumb, applying sufficient pressure to blanche the nail bed (Table 5).

The clinical course is variable and often prolonged. Many patients have considerable disability despite the lack of many physical signs, and the response to treatment is often poor.

Management
• Give advice on all the general measures of pain control (see "General Principles of Management" section).

- Advise a regular programme of exercise. Swimming is the best form of exercise, although other simple graded exercise regimes are also helpful with advice to gradually increase the amount of exercise.

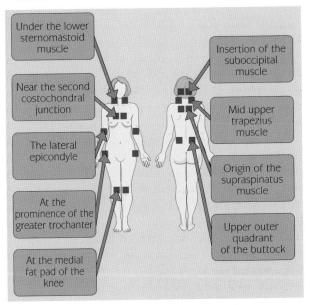

Under the lower sternomastoid muscle

Near the second costochondral junction

The lateral epicondyle

At the prominence of the greater trochanter

At the medial fat pad of the knee

Insertion of the suboccipital muscle

Mid upper trapezius muscle

Origin of the supraspinatus muscle

Upper outer quadrant of the buttock

Figure 32. The distribution of hyperalgesic points in fibromyalgia.

Diagnostic criteria for fibromyalgia[54]

1. Generalized musculo-skeletal pain and stiffness for >3 months (pain must be present on both sides of the body above and below the waist, and in the cervical, dorsal or lumbar spine)
2. Chronic fatigue and sleep disturbance
3. Tenderness of at least 11 hyperalgesic points
4. No clinical evidence of synovitis
5. Normal investigations (e.g. ESR, CRP, RhF, ANA)

Table 5. Diagnostic criteria for fibromyalgia.[54]

- Recommend a narrow (2.5-inch diameter) soft foam collar to sleep in as a therapeutic trial.
- The most effective drug therapy is one of the sedating tricyclic antidepressants, e.g. amitriptyline[53] or dothiepin in doses of 25–150 mg at night. The response to the more potent SSRIs in fibromyalgia is disappointing; it is possible that certain TCAs may partially reverse the abnormality in sleep disturbance.

Soft tissue lesions of the shoulder

Pain in the shoulder joint is more likely to be a result of a soft tissue lesion than arthritis. It is often associated with neck pain, and a specific lesion in the shoulder should be distinguished from referred pain from the cervical spine. Rotator cuff tendinitis is the commonest problem and may progress to an adhesive capsulitis or "frozen shoulder". Bicipital tendinitis, acromio-clavicular joint pain and subacromial bursitis are among the differential diagnoses. The diagnostic criteria for certain shoulder lesions are described in Table 6.

Management

- Avoid activities that exacerbate symptoms.
- Exercises:
  - Using either an ankle weight on the wrist or holding a 1 kg weight, swing the arm like a pendulum in front of the body, then side to side, allowing the arm to raise as high as possible. Repeat twice daily.
  - Wrap a weight on a walking stick and, whilst supine keep the arms straight by the sides. Holding the stick with both hands, raise the arms and let the stick fall gently above the head, then slowly return the arms to the sides. Repeat 10 times twice daily.
- Heat pack or heat lamp.
- Paracetamol with or without weak opioids.
- Therapeutic trial of NSAIDs or coxibs.
- Steroid injection (Figure 33).

Diagnostic criteria for soft tissue lesions of the shoulder[55]

Rotator cuff tendonitis: History of pain in the deltoid region and pain on resisted active movement (abduction – supraspinatus; external rotation – infraspinatus; internal rotation – subscapularis)

Bicipital tendinitis: History of anterior shoulder pain and pain on resisted active flexion or supination of the forearm

Shoulder capsulitis: History of pain in the deltoid area and equal restriction of active and passive glenohumeral movement with a capsular pattern (external rotation > abduction > internal rotation)

Table 6. Diagnostic criteria for soft tissue lesions of the shoulder.[55]

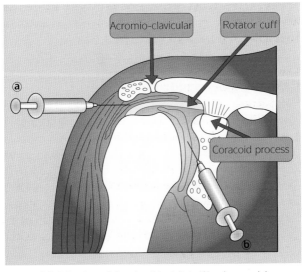

Figure 33. Injection of the shoulder joint: (A) subacromial approach; (B) anterior approach. Reproduced with kind permission of the Arthritis Research Campaign (www.arc.org.uk).

Epicondylitis

This is a common condition and can be considered to be an overuse injury. There is pain and tenderness at the insertion of the common flexor tendon over the lateral epicondyle (tennis elbow) with pain on resisted extension of the wrist, or common extensor tendon over the medial epicondyle (golfer's elbow) with pain on resisted flexion of the wrist. It often occurs in patients with coexistent cervical spondylosis.

Management
- Avoid activities that cause exacerbation.
- Symptomatic relief from ice packs.
- Try a tennis elbow splint.
- Try NSAID gel (t.i.d. for 2 weeks).
- Steroid injection (Figure 34). Infiltrate the tender area down to the periosteum with 40 mg methylprednisolone plus lignocaine. This may need to be repeated several times before there is adequate resolution of symptoms.
- Manipulation under anaesthetic for resistant cases. Surgical intervention is rarely indicated.

Carpal tunnel syndrome

This is usually ideopathic but may be associated with fluid retention, hypothyroidism or inflammatory arthritis of the wrist joint. Symptoms are variable but the diagnosis is considered in patients with pain or paraesthesiae in a median nerve distribution, particularly if nocturnal symptoms predominate. Some patients develop pain radiating up the arm that may lead to delay in diagnosis. Symptoms may be reproduced in some patients by flexing the wrist (Phalen's test) or tapping over the median nerve at the wrist (Hoffman–Tinel test). Weakness of the flexor pollicis brevis and wasting of the thenar eminence may be apparent in chronic cases. The diagnosis is confirmed with nerve conduction studies.

Management
- Symptoms may resolve spontaneously.
- Advise sleeping in a wrist splint.

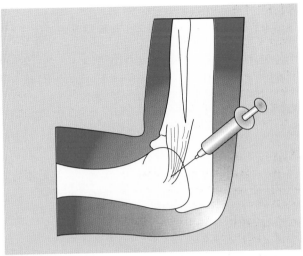

Figure 34. Injection for tennis elbow. Reproduced with kind permission of the Arthritis Research Campaign (www.arc.org.uk).

Consider an intralesional steroid injection.
- Inject the wrist joint if there is synovitis.
- Surgery is indicated if symptoms persist.

Plantar fasciitis

Pain under the heel is usually caused by plantar fasciitis, often triggered by trauma. Calcaneal spurs are a common incidental finding on X-ray, are age related, and are not usually associated with pain except when associated with sero-negative spondylo-arthropathy. Plantar fasciitis is particularly associated with Reiter's syndrome, when it has been termed "lover's heel". X-rays do not therefore usually contribute to management. Examination may be remarkably normal, with little or no tenderness despite severe symptoms, but should include the Achilles tendon to exclude symptoms from Achilles tendinitis.

Management
- Use a shock-absorbing heel pad (e.g. sorbothane).
- Inject the heel with 40 mg methylprednisolone and lignocaine. It is easier (and less traumatic) to insert the

needle into the medial side of the heel above the heel pad, rather than through the thick skin under the heel.

Repetitive strain injury (RSI)

In its true form, RSI is a tendinitis caused by repeated activity. The affected tendon will be swollen with crepitus of the tendon on passive movement of the affected digit. Infiltrating the tender area with methylprednisolone will usually improve symptoms (taking care not to inject the tendon directly). Some patients who regularly use a computer keyboard may complain of chronic pain in the hand or forearm. This is often labelled as RSI even in the absence of any abnormal signs. The pathogenesis and management in such patients is a matter of continued debate.

Bursitis

The commonest bursae to cause symptoms are those over the olecranon, the greater trochanter, the knee and the subacromial bursa. Swelling of the olecranon bursa is usually apparent. There are several bursae around the knee joints. A bursitis may develop from recurrent trauma, e.g. infra-patellar bursitis (housemaid's knee). The aetiology in many patients, however, is unclear. The diagnosis is made by the presence of a localized swelling around the patella.

Trochanteric bursitis may be associated with lumbar spondylosis, and leads to complaints of "hip pain" and difficulty in sleeping – lying on the affected side exacerbates the pain. It is often mistaken for OA of the hip, but is differentiated by the absence of groin pain, a good range of movement in the hip, and tenderness over the greater trochanter.

An intralesional steroid injection usually resolves the symptoms from a bursitis.

Hypermobility syndrome

Some patients with hypermobile joints may develop localized or generalized joint pain. For example, anterior knee pain in young adults is often caused by hypermobility of the patella tendon leading to patello-femoral dysfunction from abnormal tracking of the patella. The diagnosis is suggested by the presence of hypermobility indicated by a Carter–Wilkinson score greater than 6/9 (Table 7). Swimming and appropriate muscle strengthening exercises usually improve symptoms.

Carter–Wilkinson score of hypermobility

Score 1 for each of the following:

(a) Extension of each little finger to 90°
(b) Touch the forearm with each thumb, flexing the wrist
(c) Hyperextension of each elbow ≥190°
(d) Hyperextension of each knee ≥190°
(e) Place flat of hands on the floor while touching the toes, keeping the legs straight

Maximum score = 9

Table 7. Carter–Wilkinson score of hypermobility.

Osteoarthritis

OA is a disease of cartilage and until relatively recently was considered to be a normal consequence of ageing; it is still often referred to as degenerative joint disease. However, it has been increasingly recognized that the aetiology of OA is multifactorial, resulting from a range of factors including mechanical, inflammatory and biochemical processes in addition to genetic factors.[56, 57] OA may occur secondary to trauma and to certain congenital conditions such as epiphyseal dysplasia, but in most patients, other than a familial tendency, the cause is not apparent. Nevertheless, the strongest factors associated with OA are age and gender. Studies indicate that OA is present in more than 80% of populations over the age of 55 years and less than 0.1% of those under the age of 34 years.[58] Women are more than twice as commonly affected as men of the same age and weight.

The influence of hormonal factors is complex.[59] There is an increased incidence of nodal OA in some women a few years either side of the menopause. Unfortunately, oestrogen therapy does not appear to improve outcome.[60] In contrast, there is evidence that an increased bone density is associated with an increased risk of OA. Although there is therefore a theoretical risk of worsening OA associated with the increase in bone density from oestrogen treatment in post-menopausal women, this has not been demonstrated in clinical studies.[61, 62]

It is likely that the different patterns of OA are associated with a different aetiology. For example, obesity is associated with OA of the knee joint but not the hip. Female patients with unilateral OA have a significant risk of developing contralateral disease, and an enhanced risk is associated with increasing weight. It has been calculated that for every increase in body mass index of two units – equivalent to approximately 5 kg – there is a 1.36-fold increase in radiographic knee OA.[63] In contrast, losing weight has been found to reduce the risk of developing symptomatic OA.[64] This association appears to be not just mechanical, but to be related to the metabolic factors associated with obesity. This is supported by the association between OA in the hand and obesity. One study found more than a three-fold risk of OA in the hand in obese patients without pre-existing disease.[65] In contrast, an association between obesity and hip OA has not been found in most studies, an observation that emphasizes the aetiological complexity of OA.[66]

Different patterns of OA

The physical signs of crepitus, restricted joint movement and bony swelling are indicative of OA and may be confirmed with X-ray appearances that include joint space narrowing, sclerosis, osteophytes, cysts and joint destruction (Table 8). OA presents in a number of distinct patterns: nodal, axial, cox-arthrosis (hip) and gon-arthrosis (knee).

Nodal

The most common form of OA is termed nodal OA because of the development of Heberden's and Bouchard's nodes. These are osteophytes that cause bony swellings at the DIP and PIP joints respectively (in contrast with synovial swelling from inflammatory arthritis, which usually develops in the MCP and PIP joints and does not feel bone hard). Nodal OA also affects the CMC joints of the thumb (Figure 35) and the MTP joints of the hallux.

X-ray criteria for osteoarthritis
Joint space narrowing
Osteophytes
Subchondral sclerosis
Cysts

Table 8. X-ray criteria for OA.

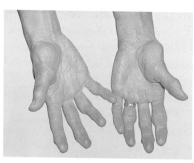

Figure 35. OA of the CMC joints of the thumbs.

Nodal OA is found in over 60% of women who have reached the age of 70 years.[58] It is less prevalent in men. OA in the CMC joints in the thumb is often painful, in contrast to Heberden's and Bouchard's nodes, which often cause some stiffness but little pain; it is more common for patients to complain of either a reduction in hand grip or the cosmetic effect from the deformity, although some patients may have pain when the nodes first develop, especially in women with peri-menopausal OA. Pain from the CMC joint of the thumb may sometimes feel as though it arises from the wrist joint, but the bony swelling of the CMC joint is usually apparent on examination, and firm pressure over the joint will reproduce the symptoms.

X-rays are not necessary to make the diagnosis but may be required to exclude either peri-articular calcification from calcium pyrophosphate disease or erosions from other inflammatory joint diseases, such as RA.

Management of nodal OA

- Reassurance – the prognosis is good.
- Avoid undue joint strain and repetitive movements.
- Advise a thumb splint for OA of the thumb CMC joint (Figure 21).
- Exercises:
  - Squeeze a small rubber ball or "play-dough" regularly through the day.
  - Pull fine threads from a ball of play-dough between the thumb and each finger individually with each hand. Repeat twice daily.

- – Make a fist and wrap an elastic band around the fingers then slowly open the hand. Repeat 10 times twice daily.
- Use hot water or hot wax bath for relief.
- Consider NSAID gel.
- Paracetamol with or without weak opioids.
- Consider therapeutic trial of NSAID or coxibs.
- Consider intralesional steroid injection.
- Surgery is rarely indicated, except for persistent pain associated with increasing deformity (usually in the thumb).

Hallux rigidus and hallux valgus are common, and are often symptomatic only with poorly designed footwear. The patient may complain of pain directly in the great toe or sometimes may have pain across the ball of the foot. The diagnosis is made by the presence of bony swelling in the MTP joint of the hallux, with fibular deviation and bunion formation in those with hallux valgus.

Management of foot pain

- Losing weight may help obese patients.
- Advice on joint protection, i.e. better footwear. High heels should be avoided and the shoe should be sufficiently broad with a cushioned sole.
- Recommend a metatarsal pad or insole.
- Valgus heel pad for pes planus with valgus of the ankle.
- Advice on simple pain control, e.g. foot baths, NSAID gels, simple analgesia.
- Refer for surgery for persistent symptoms despite the above advice.

Always advise better footwear in patients with pain in the forefoot. Shoes should be sufficiently broad with a low heel and a cushioned sole.

Axial

OA occurs almost universally in the spine in those who are middle aged or older, with a poor relation between radiographic appearances and symptoms. As the intervertebral discs degenerate, increased force is directed through the facet joints with the development of OA. Pain may arise directly from these structures and be localized to the arthritis in the spine or may result from nerve entrapment from osteophytic encroachment in the root foramina and be referred to the shoulder or pelvic region.

Patients with cervical spondylosis often complain of periscapular or shoulder pain that may be misinterpreted as disease in the shoulder joint. Similarly, patients with lumbar spondylosis frequently complain of pain in the hip, from referred pain into the gluteal region. In contrast, pain from OA of the hip joint is referred anteriorly into the groin and occasionally into the thigh or knee.

Management of cervico-brachial pain

- To avoid heavy lifting and carrying.
- Advise sleeping in a *narrow* soft collar. If intolerant try a sculpted or butterfly pillow.
- Try hot packs or heat lamp.
- Consider TENS.
- Paracetamol with or without weak opioids.
- Therapeutic trial of NSAIDs or coxibs.
- Therapeutic trial of amitryptiline or dothiepin.

Management of chronic back pain

- Advise weight reduction for obese patients.
- Avoid any heavy lifting. Advise care when travelling not to lift heavy suitcases – putting suitcases in and out of a car is a common cause of flare-up in the back.
- Avoid stooping – bend the knees or kneel on one knee "even when picking up a tea towel".
- Avoid sitting in soft armchairs and sofas.
- Use a simple lumbar support when sitting for a prolonged period of time, e.g. in an office chair (Figure 36) or car.
- Ensure the bed gives adequate support – if the bed is old, suggest either a board under the middle of the mattress or a new bed. ("Orthopaedic" beds are often too firm for

comfort – the mattress simply needs to support the normal contours of the back.)

- Consider lightweight lumbar support for heavier activity.
- Exercises:
  - Take up swimming regularly.
  - Laying prone, push up the upper body, arching the back with the pelvis on the bed or floor, then slowly lower down. Repeat five times.
  - Pelvic tilt: laying supine with knees flexed, contract abdominal muscles and flatten the low back on the bed or floor. Hold for 5 seconds and repeat five times.
  - Hip flexion: laying supine with the knees flexed, gently pull each knee in turn to the chest for 5 seconds and repeat five times for each leg.
  - Laying supine with the knees flexed, slowly roll the knees to one side and hold for 10 seconds. Repeat each side five times.
- Try hot packs or heat lamp, etc.
- Use a hot shower or bath for a flare-up.
- Consider TENS.
- Paracetamol with or without weak opioids.
- Therapeutic trial of NSAIDs or coxibs.
- Therapeutic trial of amitriptyline or dothiepin.

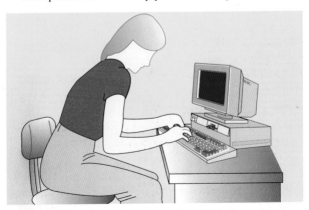

Figure 36. Poor posture whilst seated at a desk. Reproduced with kind permission of the Arthritis Research Campaign (www.arc.org.uk).

Knee

All three compartments in the knee joint may be affected with OA, although the medial compartment and patello-femoral joint are typical. Lateral compartment OA is unusual and may lead to valgus deformity, in contrast with a varus deformity from OA in the medial compartment (Figure 37).

Patients with patello-femoral OA often complain of pain with repeated flexion and extension of the knee, such as walking up or down stairs. Pain when walking on flat surfaces suggests disease in the tibio-femoral joints.

Management

- Weight reduction.
- Walking stick.
- Quads exercises:
  - Sitting back in a chair, lift one foot off the floor straightening the leg and hold it for a slow count of 10. Repeat each leg at least 10 times, and preferably throughout the day. Recommend using an ankle weight for those who are able to undertake more intensive exercise.
  - Laying supine with a rolled up towel under the heel, push the leg down firmly into the bed and hold for a slow count of 5. Repeat with each leg five times.
  - Laying supine with the leg held straight, lift the foot just off the bed and hold for a slow count of 5. Repeat with each leg five times.
- Try hot packs, etc.
- Consider TENS.
- Paracetamol with or without weak opioids.
- Therapeutic trial of NSAIDs or coxibs.
- Therapeutic trial of amytriptyline or dothiepin.
- Intra-articular steroid injection.

Intra-articular steroid injection may give symptomatic relief but is more effective when there is an effusion. The response may vary from no perceived benefit to a reduction in pain lasting for 12 months or more. The duration of response is significantly increased if the patient is completely non-weight-

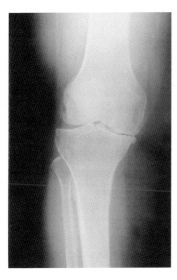

Figure 37. Medial compartment OA of the knee with joint space narrowing and osteophytes.

bearing for 24 hours after the procedure[67] – walking for even brief periods may stimulate the synovial pump, clearing the steroid from the joint more rapidly. The frequency of repeat injection is dictated by the clinical response.

For maximal response, ensure patients are completely non-weight bearing for 24 hours after an intra-articular injection into the knee joint.

Hip

OA of the hip often presents as unilateral disease but may be bilateral (Figure 38) and usually deteriorates gradually over 2–3 years, leading to hip arthroplasty.[68] Pain is the predominant symptom: initially this is related to activity, but in more advanced disease, pain at rest is an increasing problem. Nocturnal pain that wakes the patient from sleep is often used as an indication for surgery. Sleep may also be disturbed by pain from the lumbar spine and may be confused with arthritis of the hip joint if the pain is referred into the gluteal region. Remember that pain arising from the hip joint is usually felt in the groin and the anterior thigh – it is unusual for a patient

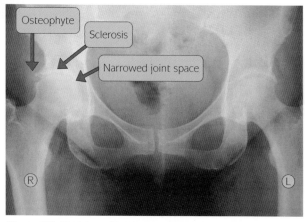

Figure 38. Moderate OA of the right hip with lesser changes on the left.

to complain of pain in the trochanteric, iliac or gluteal region arising from the hip joint, and other causes of pain should be considered.

Management

- Walking stick.
- Exercises:
  - Gentle swimming.
  - Quads exercises.
  - Swing the leg like a pendulum laterally, forwards and backwards.[11]
- Pain control as above.
- Refer for surgery if there is increasing disability and pain.

Ask patients complaining of pain in the "hip" to point to the site of pain. In the absence of groin pain, pain that is lateral or posterior to the hip is unlikely to be arising from the hip joint.

Management of Acute Synovitis

The presentation of acute synovitis is a challenging medical problem. The diagnosis may be apparent from the history. It is particularly important to determine any prodromal symptoms of a viral illness, skin rash, conjunctivitis, GI disturbance or urinary symptoms, and to enquire specifically about any past history or family history of psoriasis, iritis, inflammatory bowel disease or gout.

There may be considerable synovial swelling or joint effusions and the distribution of joint involvement is important. A monoarthritis, particularly of the knee joint, is a common feature of a sero-negative spondylo-arthritis, including reactive arthritis. A polyarthritis in a rheumatoid distribution may also occur in reactive arthritis, but may be the first presentation of RA.

Investigations may be unhelpful. If possible, aspirate a joint, particularly if there is a possibility of septic arthritis. Initial investigations should include a urine microscopy and culture, full blood count, renal and liver function tests, serum urate, ESR, CRP, and rheumatoid factor. In addition, tests for ANA and viral serology, especially for parvovirus, may be indicated. If there is a recent history of traveller's diarrhoea, then a fresh stool culture should be analysed for parasites and culture.

Whilst waiting for the results of initial investigations, treat the patient with analgesia and either an NSAID or coxib in high dose. If sepsis is excluded and there is little improvement, most patients will respond rapidly to pulse steroid – either orally (e.g. 20–30 mg daily for 5–7 days), or intramuscular methylprednisolone or triamcinolone acetonide (80 mg).

Unless there is rapid and full resolution of symptoms, refer for an urgent rheumatological opinion.

Polymyalgia Rheumatica – Diagnosis and Management

Introduction

Polymyalgia rheumatica (PMR) is a common cause of rheumatic pain in the elderly and is a condition that may be managed confidently in primary care. It occurs with increasing frequency with age, with a prevalence of almost 1% in patients over the age of 50 years.[4] It does not occur in patients under the age of 50 years and is uncommon under the age of 60 years. It is part of a spectrum of disease associated with giant cell arteritis (temporal arteritis or cranial arteritis). Symptoms of PMR occur in approximately half the patients with temporal arteritis, whereas only 15% of patients with PMR develop temporal arteritis.[69] Although antibodies have not (yet) been associated with this condition, it is useful to consider it as part of the spectrum of connective tissue diseases, particularly because of its similarity in presentation to a myalgic onset of RA.

Never make a diagnosis of PMR in a patient under the age of 50 years, and always consider other diagnoses in patients under the age of 60 years.

History

Diagnosis is usually apparent when there is a classical presentation of pain and stiffness in a symmetrical distribution in the shoulder girdle and pelvic girdle in an elderly patient.[69] There may be a sudden onset, with some patients unable to get out of bed unaided on waking one morning; others may develop increasing symptoms over several weeks. Occasionally, there may be a history of trauma that predates the onset.

Prolonged early morning stiffness is a cardinal feature of the disease, and the diagnosis should be challenged in patients without any morning stiffness. Mild depressive symptoms and sleep disturbance are common. Jaw claudication occurs in some patients and is suggestive of more severe disease or associated temporal arteritis. It is important to determine if there are any symptoms associated with temporal arteritis, including unilateral temporal headache or visual disturbance.

Systemic features including malaise, fatigue and weight loss are features of more severe disease. Some patients may also develop a low grade fever and night sweats, but if systemic features predominate then infection, malignancy and polyarteritis nodosa should be considered.

The diagnosis is more difficult in those with atypical symptoms. Some patients may have an insidious onset over several months, when symptoms may be attributed to minor trauma or to spondylosis in the cervical or lumbar spine. An asymmetrical presentation may be confused with a rotator cuff lesion in the shoulder or arthritis in the hip or spine. Peripheral joint pain is unusual but may rarely predominate and may suggest a diagnosis of RA. Carpal tunnel syndrome occurs in approximately 10% of patients and may be mistaken as the primary rather than secondary diagnosis.[70]

Clinical examination

The physical signs are usually subtle. Stiffness is often apparent during physical examination. The patients may have an abnormal gait, and have difficulty climbing onto the examination couch or rising from a chair. Many patients will have minor tenderness in the proximal muscle groups, but *muscle power is normal*. However, the patient may be reluctant to assist with the examination because of muscle stiffness.

Clinical examination may be normal, and other diagnoses must be considered in patients with definite muscle weakness.

Restriction in the range of movement of joints is usually mild and may only be found in those with more severe disease. A mild degree of synovial swelling may be present in the knees and wrists and occasionally in the MCP joints,[70] but if synovial swelling is prominent, the diagnosis is more likely to be RA or other inflammatory joint disease. Formal examination of the joints may be remarkably normal and may suggest the diagnosis in a patient with significant symptoms.

It is important to examine the temporal arteries in all patients. Look at the temple for any prominence of the artery, and palpate both arteries for any thickening or tenderness. Ensure that the pulse is present in both arteries. Any tenderness or localized thickening of the arterial wall or an absent pulse should be considered to be a sign of temporal arteritis. (Any patient with suspected temporal arteritis should be commenced on treatment and referred to a rheumatologist.)

Investigations

The characteristic finding in PMR is a raised acute phase response. The results may be considerably raised in some patients. However, a minority of patients do not have an elevated acute phase, often leading to difficulty in diagnosis.[71] Anaemia of chronic disease is found more commonly in those with systemic symptoms. Mild elevation of hepatic trans-aminases is common. Muscle enzymes are always normal. Auto-antibodies are not associated with PMR or temporal arteritis; a positive rheumatoid factor would suggest a myalgic onset of RA.

A positive biopsy of the temporal artery is diagnostic of temporal arteritis, but the vascular abnormalities are patchy and a negative biopsy does not exclude this diagnosis.[71] A temporal artery biopsy is therefore usually only undertaken in patients with unusual symptoms and signs.

Steroid trial

A characteristic feature of PMR is a rapid response to steroids. The majority of patients will have a significant and often complete remission with a dose of 20–30 mg daily of prednisolone. A response is usually seen within 24 hours with complete resolution of symptoms within a week.

The response in patients with severe disease is one of the most remarkable in medicine. Patients who may have been significantly disabled with pain and stiffness for several weeks or months appear to be "cured" within days. If there is a poor response this usually implies another diagnosis, although a minority of patients may need either a higher dose or non-coated tablets to improve absorption. Higher doses need to be used in temporal arteritis – if steroids are prescribed as a therapeutic trial in patients with unilateral headache, it is advisable to use doses up to 60 mg daily.

Always check the FBC, ESR, CRP, CK and rheumatoid factor before prescribing a therapeutic trial of steroids. A normal ESR and CRP does not exclude mild PMR, but an elevated CK indicates myopathy or myositis. A high titre of rheumatoid factor suggests RA.

Differential diagnosis

The differential diagnosis of PMR includes early RA and fibromyalgia. A myalgic onset of RA may be indistinguishable from PMR, and the diagnosis is often made because of a strongly positive rheumatoid factor or the subsequent clinical course. Fibromyalgia is unusual in the elderly, but may occasionally be confused with mild PMR without an acute phase response. Soft tissue lesions of the shoulder may also be confused with atypical PMR, but the lack of a dramatic response to a trial of steroids is a useful guide to the non-specialist. Some patients with cervical and lumbar spondylosis may also have diffuse symptoms that may be confused with mild PMR, but similarly would not have a dramatic response to a steroid trial.

PMR can usually be recognized as distinct from polymyositis and proximal myopathies because of the almost universal finding of muscle weakness in these conditions. Check the thyroid and renal function, calcium, potassium and other biochemistry if a myopathy is suspected. Malignancies (including lymphomas and myeloma) should always be considered in those with systemic symptoms.

Management

Corticosteroids are the only effective treatment and are continued until there is a natural remission of the disease. The dosage and duration of treatment in patients with temporal arteritis are approximately double those for PMR. In most patients with PMR, treatment is continued for a minimum of 12 months, although many patients may not be able to tail off treatment for 2 years or more.[72] A minority of patients are unable to tail off steroids and remain on chronic treatment. The dosage is gradually reduced over time and should be the minimum that completely abolishes the symptoms. The dosage should be dictated by the patient's symptoms and response to treatment; the ESR and CRP should also influence the steroid dose in temporal arteritis. In comparison with the CRP, the ESR is subject to wide variation and is a poor guide to disease activity in PMR.[73]

Recommend the lowest steroid doses that maintain full clinical remission for the duration of the disease. Use symptoms rather than ESR as a guide to dose in PMR, and a combination of symptoms and ESR or CRP in temporal arteritis.

Many patients prefer to tolerate minor symptoms in order to take a lower dose of steroids. It is advisable to warn against doing so, as it is rarely possible to tail off steroids unless a complete remission is sustained for at least 12 months, and those who take too low a dose often remain on treatment for several years. Except when large doses cause dyspepsia and need to be divided, it is more physiological and causes less side-effects for treatment to be taken in a single dose with breakfast.[74]

Treatment regimes

There are a number of regimes that have been advocated. A regime that is usually effective for mild or moderate disease is given in Table 9. Using such an alternate day regime has some theoretical advantages in causing fewer side-effects than equivalent daily doses[75] and may be slightly more effective. The

A treatment regime for polymyalgia rheumatica

EC Prednisolone

20 mg daily for 2 weeks,
15 mg daily for 2 weeks,
15 and 10 mg alternate days for 2 weeks,
10 mg daily for 2 weeks,
10 and 5 mg alternate days for 3 months,
5 mg daily for 6 months,
then attempt to tail off
(e.g. 5 and 2.5 mg alternate days for 1 month,
2.5 mg daily for 1 month,
2.5 mg alternate days for 1 month, then discontinue)

Table 9. A treatment regime for polymyalgia rheumatica.

duration of any one dose in this regime should be prolonged if there is a recurrence of symptoms. If symptoms recur, double the dose for 1 week then reduce to the previous lowest effective dose for approximately 3 months before attempting further dose reduction. For example, if symptoms recur after reducing from 10 mg daily to alternate 10 and 5 mg, then increase to 15 mg daily for 1 week, then reduce to 10 mg daily for 3 months, before reducing again to alternate doses of 10 and 5 mg daily.

Patients with mild disease, i.e. those with normal or only slightly raised CRP at diagnosis, should be able to tail off treatment after 12 months. In those with more severe disease presenting with considerable elevation of acute phase proteins, anaemia or systemic features, the dose regime will need to be prolonged. For example, if there is a relapse with reduction to 10 mg daily after 6 weeks, continue alternate 15/10 mg for 1–3 months, then reduce to 10 mg daily for 3 months, reducing to 10/5 mg daily for 6 months before reducing to 5 mg daily.

A suggested regime for temporal arteritis is to double both the doses and duration of this regime, e.g. 40 mg daily for 4 weeks, then 30 mg daily for 4 weeks, etc. However, if the ESR or CRP are not suppressed in patients with temporal arteritis, it is advisable to increase the dose of treatment appropriately in view of the potential risk of sudden blindness.

In those who are resistant to treatment and need sustained high doses of steroids, consider using azathioprine or methotrexate as a "steroid-sparing agent". Side-effects are relatively common; start on 50 mg daily of azathioprine and increase to 100–150 mg daily dependent on body weight. For methotrexate, there is not as much experience and the choice of dose seems to be governed by an empiric approach. The dose should probably not be higher than 20-25 mg once per week and the initial doses should begin at about 15 mg per week. Folic acid should be administered concomitantly.

Monitor for potential side-effects of steroids as discussed in the "Drug Treatment" section.

Gout and Other Crystal Diseases

Gout is a common disease that is often managed fully in primary care. It can be categorized as either primary or secondary, and either acute or chronic (tophaceous). Primary gout is one of the most common inherited defects of metabolism, causing impaired purine metabolism and hyperuricaemia.[76]

It occurs predominantly in men. It may also occur in postmenopausal women, when it is often secondary to thiazide and occasionally loop diuretics.[77]

Acute gout

The diagnosis of gout should be considered in all cases of acute monoarthritis. Pain and swelling of the affected joint are universal features of acute gout. The severity of pain may suggest the diagnosis – only septic arthritis is likely to be more painful. In some patients, even the weight of bedding may be intolerable, and the symptoms may be so intense that the vibration of someone walking across the room may exacerbate the pain. Erythema is a common physical sign in acute gout and is uncommon in most other forms of arthritis other than septic arthritis and (occasionally) reactive arthritis.

The MTP joint of the hallux is most commonly affected in acute gout; the majority of patients with gout will develop an acute attack in this joint. The characteristic clinical appearance of severe pain, swelling and erythema in the first MTP joint is termed "podagra" and the association of podagra with hyperuricaemia is diagnostic of gout (Figure 39). However, most other joints may be affected with gout, although it is doubtful whether it occurs in the hip joints or facet joints. The forefoot, ankle and knee are commonly affected; less commonly affected are the small joints of the hands, the wrists, elbows and shoulder joints (Figure 40). Joints that have pre-existing arthritis are often affected (OA of the first MTP joint is almost universal

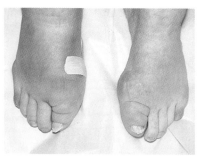

Figure 39. Acute podagra.

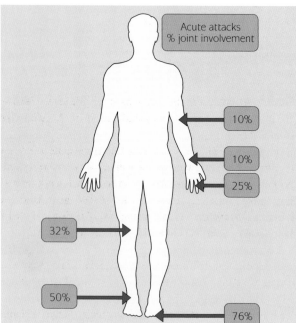

Acute attacks
% joint involvement

10%

10%

25%

32%

50%

76%

Figure 40. Incidence of acute gout in different joints. Reproduced with permission from BMJ Publishing Group from Grahame R. Scott JT. *Ann Rheum Dis* 1970; **29**: 461–468.[78]

and may be an explanation for the predisposition of gout in this joint). Acute bursitis, particularly of the olecranon bursa, may occur in some patients. Less commonly, gout may cause a polyarthritis, when the diagnosis may be more problematic.

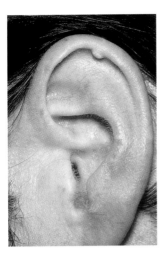

Figure 41. Gouty tophus on the pinna.

Always look for tophi in any patient with acute arthritis, as their presence is a strong indication of the diagnosis (Figure 41).

Hyperuricaemia is usual, at least during an acute attack, but occasionally the uric acid may be within the normal range, and is often normal in between attacks. In addition, hyperuricaemia is not uncommon in patients who do not have gout. Uric acid is excreted by the kidney and the majority of patients with renal failure have hyperuricaemia without developing gout.

A normal uric acid does not exclude gout, and a raised uric acid is not diagnostic.

The most important differential diagnosis is sepsis – either a septic arthritis or cellulitis. Systemic features such as malaise and fever associated with a leukocytosis and raised acute phase response do not necessarily indicate sepsis, as they may also occur in severe attacks of gout. Unless the diagnosis of gout is certain, joint aspiration is mandatory. The synovial fluid in acute gout may have the appearance of pus due to the intensity of inflammation causing a florid neutrophil response, but a definitive diagnosis of gout is made by demonstrating intracellular sodium mono-urate crystals (Figure 42) that are

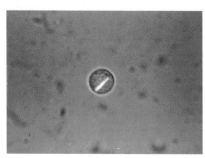

Figure 42.
Intracellular sodium mono-urate crystal.

negatively birefringent on polarizing microscopy (Table 10). If there is any doubt, it is preferable to initiate antibiotics *after* aspiration whilst waiting for culture.

Antibiotics should never be prescribed for a possible diagnosis of septic arthritis without arranging synovial fluid culture.

Differential diagnosis of acute gout

In addition to sepsis, a stress fracture in the forefoot may be mistaken for podagra. Other forms of inflammatory arthritis may be mistaken for gout. Acute pseudo-gout is more common in the elderly and attacks typically affect the knee or wrist. The degree of inflammation is usually mild, although there may be some erythema. Reactive arthritis, including Reiter's syndrome, may occasionally cause intense inflammation with systemic symptoms and localized erythema, swelling and severe pain, and may be difficult to differentiate from acute gout. It is uncommon for the severity of inflammation to be as intense in other forms of inflammatory arthritis, but a mild attack of gout may resemble a monoarthritis from RA or psoriatic arthritis.

Treatment of an acute attack

An acute attack of gout will usually respond rapidly to a full dose of any anti-inflammatory drug. This treatment may also be used in the elderly providing the treatment period is limited to a few days. However, if there is a contraindication to an NSAID, large doses of a coxib should be as effective.

Diagnostic criteria for gout
Urate crystals in synovial fluid
A previous history of podagra
The presence of tophi
Hyperuricaemia
Rapid response to colchicine

Table 10. Diagnostic criteria for gout.

An alternative is to prescribe colchicine. A major side-effect is nausea and diarrhoea, and it is almost an inevitable consequence of high doses. One regime is for a 0.5 mg dose to be repeated every 2–4 hours until resolution of symptoms or the development of diarrhoea. However, a dose of 0.5 mg t.i.d. is usually well tolerated and, although the response may not be as rapid, it can usually be continued without causing diarrhoea. Intra-articular corticosteroids may also be considered when response to drug therapy is protracted. In resistant cases, a combination of high dose NSAID plus colchicine is nearly always successful, although treatment may need to be continued for several weeks.

In an average attack, the maximal severity is usually reached over several hours and complete resolution of the earliest attacks will typically occur within a few days to several weeks, even without treatment. Resolution of the acute gouty attack is sometimes accompanied by desquamation of the skin overlying the affected joint.

Acute cutaneous tophi

There may be an acute onset of subcutaneous tophi (Figure 43) often in elderly women treated with diuretics, particularly thiazides. They often occur in the pulp of the terminal phalanx and may be intensely painful. There is whitish/yellow subcutaneous material that is exquisitely tender associated with significant hyperuricaemia. If there is any discharge of the material, the diagnosis can be confirmed with polarizing

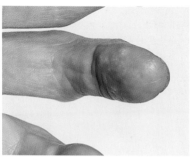

Figure 43. Acute gouty tophi.

microscopy. Treatment with colchicine may reduce the acute symptoms, but thiazide diuretics should be discontinued. Most patients will respond to a course of allopurinol.

Chronic (tophaceous) gout

Some patients have a chronic course with persistent pain and swelling, and either clusters of attacks with little or no pain free intervals, or develop polyarthritis with deposition of tophi (Figure 44). Polyarticular gout may have a similar clinical appearance to RA, particularly if there is swelling in the MCP and PIP joints. Gouty tophi in the olecranon bursae may also be mistaken for rheumatoid nodules. X-rays will usually help to differentiate: the features of gout include calcification in the joint capsule and erosions that appear to be "punched out", in contrast to the "bite-like" marginal erosions of RA. All patients with polyarticular gout or tophi should usually be treated with allopurinol.

Common sites of tophi are the pinna, extensor surfaces of the elbows, particularly in the olecranon bursae, and in the foot around the first MTP joint. In chronic cases, tophi may develop in the DIP joints and occasionally in any of the other joints in the hands.

Prevention

Any aetiological factors should be determined. Alcohol abuse is a common triggering factor. During an attack there should be complete abstention, and those with recurrent attacks should be advised to abstain fully. In other patients they should be

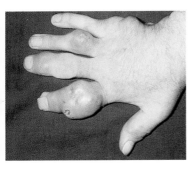

Figure 44. Chronic tophaceous gout.

advised to limit alcohol consumption to a maximum of 3 or 4 units daily.

Diuretics are a common cause of (secondary) gout.[79] Thiazides should be avoided in all patients with gout. (Ensure that hypertensive patients do not have a fixed combination drug with a small dose of a thiazide diuretic.)

Trauma and starvation may precipitate an acute attack of gout. Major trauma including surgery may cause an increase in serum uric acid, but minor trauma to the foot may trigger an attack of podagra in an individual with a predisposition to gout.

The rapid rise in serum uric acid from chemotherapy or radiotherapy for lymphoma or leukaemia may cause acute polyarticular gout and is an indication for prophylactic treatment.

Chronic hyperuricaemia may lead to renal calculi or urate nephropathy. It is advisable to monitor renal function in all patients with a significantly raised uric acid, but further discussion of these conditions is outside the scope of this book.

Allopurinol

Allopurinol is the most effective drug for the treatment of gout. It is an inhibitor of xanthine oxidase – the final step in purine metabolism, producing uric acid from xanthine.[80] It will reduce the frequency and severity of attacks, but is only effective for prophylaxis and should not be prescribed during an acute attack. The indications for treatment with allopurinol include those with recurrent acute attacks and for chronic tophaceous gout (Table 11).

Indications for allopurinol
1. Recurrent acute attacks
2. Tophaceous gout
3. Renal stones with hyperuricaemia
4. Marked hyperuricaemia with renal impairment
5. Chemotherapy or radiotherapy for lymphoma or leukaemia

Table 11. Indications for allopurinol.

Allopurinol may precipitate an acute attack and the dose should always be titrated upwards. Start on 100 mg o.d. for 1 week then 200 mg o.d. for the second week, then 300 mg o.d., except in renal failure. The active metabolite, oxypurinol, accumulates in renal failure and is nephrotoxic. For those with mild impairment (creatinine = 120–200 mmol/l), the maximum dose should be 200 mg daily, and in established renal failure (creatinine clearance less than 30 ml/min, creatinine > 200 mmol/l) should be 100 mg daily. Concomitant treatment with colchicine (0.5 mg b.i.d or t.i.d.) for the first 3 weeks of treatment will usually eliminate the risk of a treatment-induced flare.

Some patients stop the allopurinol if initiation of treatment induces a flare. It is important to warn the patient of the potential risk of a flare and treat the attack appropriately, but *not to stop treatment if it occurs* as a flare-up may develop every time the patient starts treatment.

- Allopurinol is not indicated following the first attack of gout or if attacks are very infrequent, and should never be initiated during an acute attack.
- Always start on 100 mg daily and gradually increase the dose.
- Consider concomitant treatment with colchicine during initiation of treatment to prevent a treatment-induced flare.

The response to allopurinol is impressive. For those who fail to respond, failure of compliance should be considered. Those who continue to abuse alcohol or remain on thiazide diuretics may also fail to respond. The major problem in the treatment of gout is in those who are intolerant of allopurinol. Skin rash is relatively common and may lead to withdrawal of treatment. Blood dyscrasias, GI side-effects or a hypersensitivity syndrome are uncommon, but may lead to drug withdrawal.[81] Uricosuric drugs such as probenecid are an alternative, but are usually less effective. Chronic treatment with colchicine is inadvisable because of the risk of neuromyopathy.[82]

Refer to a rheumatologist if there is intolerance or failure to respond to allopurinol.

Pseudo-gout (chondrocalcinosis, pyrophosphate arthropathy)

There are a range of clinical presentations from calcium pyrophosphate crystal deposition disease (CPPD).[83] These range from an acute attack of pseudo-gout to a rapidly destructive arthritis similar to a neuropathic or Charcot joint (although in view of the inconsistent finding of pyrophosphate crystals, this condition has also been termed apatite-associated arthritis, as hydroxyapatite is found in the synovial fluid in all patients). However, the majority of patients with CPPD are asymptomatic. The appearance of calcification in the articular cartilage is often an incidental finding on X-ray and is associated with OA. Valgus deformity of the knee may be more common in OA associated with chondrocalcinosis and some patients develop a low grade synovitis of the small joints of the hands, often associated with changes of nodal OA.

Pseudo-gout causes acute or sub-acute attacks of monoarthritis, usually affecting the knee or wrist joint, in elderly patients. The appearances may mimic acute gout with erythema and severe pain, although the inflammation is often not as severe. The attack may cause considerable soft tissue erythema and may be mistaken for a bacterial cellulitis. The diagnosis is made from synovial fluid examination with the identification of intracellular calcium pyrophosphate crystals (Figure 45). Treatment is similar to acute gout.

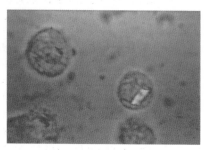

Figure 45.
Intracellular calcium pyrophosphate crystal.

Rheumatoid Arthritis

RA is the commonest inflammatory joint disease, with a prevalence of over 1%.[84] The presenting features and course of the disease vary from an individual with disease that is so mild that they never consult a doctor to someone with rapid destruction of joints or a life-threatening illness. The age of presentation varies from infancy to the very elderly, but the peak age of onset is in early middle age. Women are two to three times more commonly affected than men. The diagnosis is made largely on clinical grounds, particularly as investigations may be normal at onset and in mild disease may be normal throughout the course of the illness. The onset is usually insidious, but some patients have an acute onset.[85] The presence of significant disability at the onset of symptoms is indicative of a poor prognosis and an increased mortality (Figure 46).[86]

Although joint pain is the predominant symptom in RA,[87] in common with other inflammatory joint diseases, most patients have prolonged morning stiffness and the duration of morning stiffness is a guide to the activity of the disease. The usual presentation is with a symmetrical polyarthritis, although the disease rarely causes a "mirror image" of one side of the body to the other.[88] The symmetrical nature of the disease is an indication that similar joints tend to be affected on both sides of the body, e.g. *some* MCP joints but not necessarily the same joints. The degree of synovitis and subsequent deformity is often asymmetrical.

In established disease, approximately 90% of patients have synovitis in the hands, wrists and feet.[89] The MCP joints are usually involved, with or without the PIPs. The DIP joints are usually spared, but most of the large joints may also be affected (Figure 47). Other joints that are occasionally affected include the sterno-clavicular, acromio-clavicular and tempero-mandibular joints.[90] The hip joints and spine may also be affected in established disease (Figure 48).

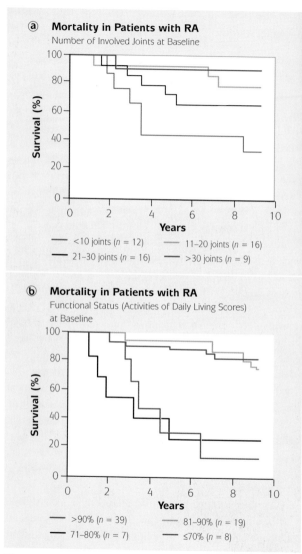

Figure 46. Mortality in patients with RA. Reproduced with permission from Pincus T, Callahan LF. *Scand J Rheumatol* 1989; **79**(Suppl): 67–96.[86]

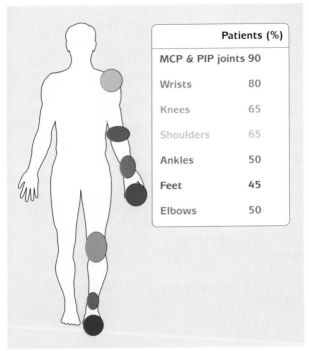

	Patients (%)
MCP & PIP joints	90
Wrists	80
Knees	65
Shoulders	65
Ankles	50
Feet	45
Elbows	50

Figure 47. Joint involvement in early RA.

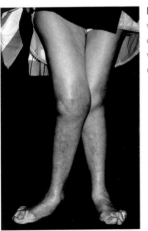

Figure 48. Severe RA with valgus deformity of the knees and ankles, hallux valgus and cock-up toe deformity.

The diagnosis is suggested by the presence of joint swelling in both hands, particularly in the MCP and PIP joints, and wrists (see Figure 5).

Rheumatoid nodules are very uncommon in early disease, but are diagnostic of RA. A raised acute phase response (ESR, plasma viscosity or CRP) is suggestive of an inflammatory arthritis, and a strongly positive rheumatoid factor in a patient with synovitis is virtually diagnostic of RA (Table 13). Both indicate a worse outcome when present at the onset of symptoms.[91, 92]

Radiographic erosions present early in the disease also indicate a poor prognosis (Table 12). Erosive changes in a rheumatoid distribution on X-ray confirm the diagnosis, although they may not occur until late in the disease. Erosions may be present in the MTP joints in patients without pain in the feet, and if RA is suspected it is therefore advisable to X-ray the feet as well as the hands (see Figure 18).

Indicators of poor prognosis in early disease

1. Female gender
2. Marked disability
3. Strongly positive rheumatoid factor
4. Raised CRP
5. Erosions on X-ray of hands or feet

Table 12. Indicators of poor prognosis in early disease.

Unusual types of presentation

Systemic

An acute onset of polyarthritis may be associated with prominent myalgia, fatigue, low grade fever, weight loss and depression. This occurs to some degree in up to a third of patients. Occasionally, the systemic features may predominate, with a clinical appearance suggestive of malignancy. In the absence of synovitis, the diagnosis may become one of exclusion and confirmed only with the development of articular disease.

Myalgic

Some patients present with symptoms that are indistinguishable from PMR. The diagnosis is suggested if there is a positive rheumatoid factor, and if peripheral arthritis develops during the course of the illness.

Palindromic rheumatism

The arthritis is episodic with either a monoarthritis or a polyarthritis lasting for hours to days. The differential diagnosis includes gout and reactive arthritis. After a prolonged follow-up, many patients develop persistent synovitis indistinguishable from those with typical RA.[88]

Monoarthritis

Approximately 10% of patients present with a monoarthritis. The knee is most commonly affected but other large joints may be involved. (Consider psoriatic arthritis if there is a monoarthritis of one of the small joints in the hand.) The majority of those with a monoarticular onset will develop a polyarthritis over subsequent weeks or months.

Carpal tunnel syndrome

The first manifestation of RA may be carpal tunnel syndrome caused by subclinical synovitis or tenosynovitis in the wrist.[93] The diagnosis is usually evident over a period of months, with the development of synovial swelling in a rheumatoid distribution.

Extra-articular disease

Rarely, the first sign of the disease is an extra-articular manifestation. Rheumatoid nodules may predate articular disease. If they occur in the lung, a nodule may be mistaken for malignancy until a biopsy is taken. Pericarditis or a rheumatoid pleural effusion developing before other signs of the disease may cause difficulty in diagnosis. Very rarely, other features including vasculitis (Figure 49), episcleritis or other ocular manifestations of RA may be the first sign of the disease, but usually develop during the course of severe sero-positive disease.

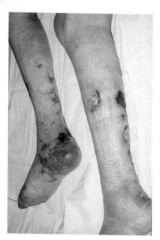

Figure 49. Severe rheumatoid vasculitis.

Clinical course

The course of the disease varies considerably. In general, those with poor prognostic indicators have persistent disease and disability unless they respond to disease-modifying anti-rheumatoid drug (DMARD) therapy. Some patients with the most severe disease have a relentless progression of joint pain and destruction without response to treatment. Conversely, some patients may have trivial disease with full resolution of symptoms and signs without a recurrence.

RA shows a marked variation of clinical expression in individual patients. This difference may be apparent in the number and pattern of joint involvement. As an example, some patients may have mainly small joints or large joints affected. Some patients may have only a few and others almost all joints involved. A subset of patients may have prominent extra-articular disease.

Management

The management of RA is determined by the degree of active synovitis. Patients with mild disease who have few symptoms, little synovitis and no risk factors are treated symptomatically as described in the section on "General Principles of Management". DMARDs are ineffective when symptoms are

American Rheumatism Association revised criteria for classification of RA

Criterion	Description
Morning stiffness	Morning stiffness in and around the joints, lasting at least 1 hour before maximal improvement.
Arthritis of three or more joint areas	At least three joint areas (out of 14 possible areas; right or left PIP, MCP, wrist, elbow, knee, ankle, MTP joints) simultaneously have had soft tissue swelling or fluid (not bony overgrowth alone) as observed by a physician.
Arthritis of hand joints	At least one area swollen in a wrist, MCP or PIP joint.
Symmetric arthritis	Simultaneous involvement of the same joint areas (as defined above) on both sides of the body (bilateral involvement of PIPs, MCPs or MTP joints without absolute symmetry is acceptable).
Rheumatoid nodules	Subcutaneous nodules over bony prominences or extensor surfaces, or in juxta-articular regions, as observed by a physician.
Serum rheumatoid factor	Demonstration of abnormal amounts of serum rheumatoid factor by any method for which the result has been positive in less than 5% of normal control subjects.
Radiographic changes	Radiographic changes typical of RA on postero-anterior hand or wrist radiographs, which must include erosions or unequivocal bony decalcification localized in, or most marked adjacent to, the involved joints (OA changes alone do not qualify).

Note: For classification purposes, a patient has RA if at least four of these criteria are satisfied (the first four must have been present for at least 6 weeks).

Table 13. American Rheumatism Association revised criteria for classification of RA.

a result of secondary OA from previous joint damage, but those with definite synovitis need to be treated with a DMARD, which should be initiated by a rheumatologist. In addition, most patients with active disease will also need to continue with simple analgesics, NSAIDs, physical treatment and exercises. Corticosteroids are an important adjunct to treatment either for intra-articular injections, as oral or intramuscular pulse therapy for flare-ups and initiation of a DMARD, or chronic low dose oral steroids for systemic disease, including anaemia and weight loss.

Disease-modifying anti-rheumatoid drugs (DMARDs; slow-acting anti-rheumatoid or "second line" drugs)

Drug treatment is usually initiated by a rheumatologist as the indications for treatment depend on accurate assessment of disease activity. DMARDs are only effective when there is active synovitis and the response is always slow. There is little observable effect within the first weeks of treatment and it is unwise to conclude that there is a failure of response until treatment is continued for a minimum of 3–4 months. Toxicity is common and it is necessary to monitor for the development of side-effects.

There is considerable individual variation in response to these drugs and also in the development of side-effects. This often leads to several drugs being prescribed in any one patient, either sequentially or in combination. The order in which each drug is prescribed varies between different rheumatologists, but is largely related to the balance between efficacy and toxicity. Although there is evidence that patients remain on methotrexate longer than other drugs, this may be explained in part by the longer dose titration with this drug, in contrast with the fixed dose of most other DMARDs (Figure 50).[94]

Hydroxychloroquine

This drug is often used in early or mild disease or in patients with a connective tissue disease. It has largely replaced chloroquine as it is better tolerated. Skin rashes may occur,

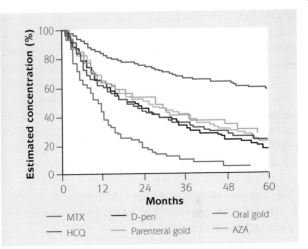

Figure 50. Rate of continuation of DMARD therapy of RA. AZA, azathioprine; D-pen, D-penicillamine; HCQ, hydroxychloroquine; MTX, methotrexate. Reproduced with permission from Pincus T, Marcum SB, Callahan LF. *J Rheumatol* 1992; **19**(12): 1885–1894.[94]

including photosensitive rashes. There is a small risk of the drug being deposited in the macula with long-term administration, although this is thought to be less common with hydroxychloroquine than chloroquine. If treatment is continued for more than 1–2 years, regular ophthalmological assessment is recommended.[95–97] The usual dose is 200 mg b.i.d., often reducing to 200 mg o.d. after clinical response. Blood monitoring is not required.

Except in exceptional circumstances, it is contraindicated to continue treatment with hydroxychloroquine for more than 5 years because of the risk of irreversible maculopathy.

Sulphasalazine (Salazopyrin)

This is considered to be the DMARD of first choice by many rheumatologists. The dose is usually built up sequentially over the first 4 weeks of treatment in order to reduce the incidence of GI upset and mild neurological symptoms, including headaches and dizziness. Some patients are unable to tolerate even small doses of the drug because of these side-effects.[98] Skin rashes are uncommon, but it may be possible to desensitize the patient with rashes by starting on a very low dose. Blood dyscrasias and hepatic dysfunction are uncommon; macrocytosis is seen occasionally and reflects the effect of sulphasalazine as a folate antagonist.

The standard regime is: week 1 – 500 mg o.d.; week 2 – 500 mg b.i.d.; week 3 – 500 mg t.i.d.; week 4 – 1 g b.i.d.

It is standard management to monitor blood count and liver function tests monthly for the first 3 months of treatment. Thereafter, side-effects are rare.

Methotrexate

Some rheumatologists consider methotrexate to be the drug of first choice for active RA.[99, 100]

Although many patients are concerned at the concept of being prescribed a drug used for "chemotherapy", serious side-effects are remarkably uncommon. There is a small risk of agranulocytosis or other haematological dyscrasias and the risk of infections is slightly increased. The most common side-effect is hepatic toxicity, with a rise in liver transaminases. With chronic use the drug may rarely lead to hepatic fibrosis and cirrhosis, although the incidence of hepatic side-effects is reduced with co-administration of folic acid. Headache and GI disturbance may cause withdrawal of treatment, although may be reduced by subcutaneous rather than oral administration.

The major concern is a hypersensitivity pneumonitis, which is a rare but potentially fatal complication.[101] This occurs in less than 1% of patients, but leads rapidly to respiratory failure and adult respiratory distress syndrome. Initial radiographic appearances include scattered fluffy white shadows. Treatment with large doses of steroids will usually prevent death if given sufficiently early and should lead to full recovery. Patients may present initially with an unexplained cough or dyspnoea; it is therefore important that patients with respiratory symptoms taking methotrexate should have a chest X-ray and be monitored closely.

Methotrexate is prescribed as a single, once weekly dose. Folic acid should be co-prescribed throughout treatment – either 5 mg weekly taken 3 or 4 days after the methotrexate or 1 mg daily except on the day of methotrexate dosing.

The starting dose is 7.5–10 mg weekly, and is increased in 2.5–5 mg increments if there is an inadequate response, up to a maximum dose of 25–30 mg weekly. A standard regime of monitoring is to measure blood count and liver enzymes weekly for the first month, fortnightly for the second month, then monthly thereafter. Patients should be urged to limit their alcohol intake while taking methotrexate.

Leflunomide (Arava)

Leflunomide is the most recent oral DMARD to be licensed for the treatment of RA. It has been studied in comparison with sulphasalazine and methotrexate in large trials (Figure 51).[102–105] The results indicate that leflunomide is at least as effective as the comparator drugs. The dose is 10 or 20 mg daily. Initiation of treatment with a loading dose (100 mg o.d. for 3 days) may give a more rapid response, but may also increase the incidence of side-effects. Response is usually seen within 6 weeks.

Serious side-effects have been rare, but there is a risk of diarrhoea in up to 20% of patients. A list of the frequency of side-effects of leflunomide, methotrexate and sulphasalazine is given in Table 14. Careful monitoring of liver transaminases and blood counts are important at a schedule similar to that described with methotrexate. Patients on either drug need to understand that they should not become pregnant while taking this therapy.

Sodium aurothiomalate (Myocrisin)

Gold salts have been used in the treatment of RA for over 50 years, but their use is declining. One of the major disadvantages is the need for the drug to be given by

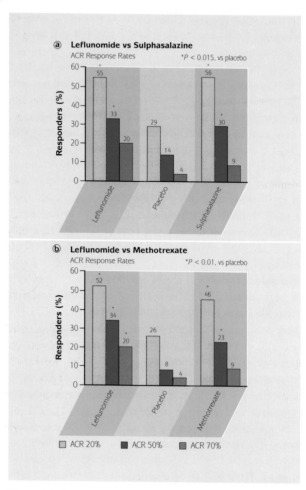

Figure 51. Response rates of leflunomide vs other DMARDs, expressed as the American College of Rheumatology (ACR) criteria based on a 20%, 50% or 70% improvement in a number of parameters, including swollen and tender joint counts, global scores and CRP. Part A reproduced with permission from Elsevier Science (The Lancet, 1999; **353**: 259.).[103] Part B used data from Strand V et al. Arch Intern Med 1999; **159**: 2542.[104]

intramuscular injection. The standard regime is to have weekly injections for approximately 20 weeks or until the patient goes into remission, at which point the frequency of injections is reduced.

The commonest side-effect of gold injections is a psoriasiform skin rash.[106, 107] This occurs more frequently with increasing total dosage. Patients can sometimes be managed by reducing the dose, but often the drug needs to be withdrawn. Blood dyscrasias are less common. Thrombocytopenia is the commonest abnormality. The drug may also cause a membranous glomerulonephritis, leading to proteinuria and eventually nephrotic syndrome if treatment is not withdrawn. A 24-hour urine collection for protein needs to be undertaken if there is more than a trace of proteinuria and the drug withdrawn if the proteinuria is significant. All patients should be monitored indefinitely with a blood count and urinalysis prior to each injection.

D-Penicillamine (Distamine)

Penicillamine used to be used widely, but it is now prescribed infrequently because of the higher incidence of side-effects. Skin rash and loss of taste may occur early during treatment.[107] Thrombocytopenia and other blood dyscrasias, and proteinuria from membranous nephropathy occur more commonly than with gold injections. Patients need to be monitored indefinitely with blood count and urinalysis, initially weekly but increasing to monthly after 3 months of treatment.

Auranofin (Ridaura)

Auranofin is an oral gold preparation with mild disease-modifying activity. Blood dyscrasia and proteinuria are very uncommon, but it is prescribed infrequently because of a high frequency of diarrhoea and relatively poor efficacy.

Azathioprine (Imuran)

Azathioprine is used most frequently in patients with evidence of systemic involvement or vasculitis. It is also prescribed as a "steroid-sparing drug" in an attempt to control inflammatory

Tolerability profile of sulphasalazine, methotrexate			
	Placebo controlled		
Adverse event	**LEF** (*n* = 315)	**PL** (*n* = 210)	**SSZ** (*n* = 133)
Gastrointestinal			
Diarrhoea	26.7	11.9	9.8
Nausea	13.0	11.0	18.8
Dyspepsia	10.2	10.0	9.0
Hepatic			
Elevated LFT	10.2	2.4	3.8
CNS			
Headache	13.3	11.4	12.0
Cardiovascular			
Hypertension	8.9	4.3	3.8
Respiratory infection	21.0	20.5	20.3
Skin			
Rash	12.4	6.7	10.5
Alopecia	8.9	1.4	6.0

LEF, leflunomide; MTX, methotrexate; PL, placebo; SSZ, sulphasala
Data taken from references 102–105.

Table 14. Tolerability profile of sulphasalazine, methotrexate and lef unomide

| | Active controlled | | All trials |
TX n = 182)	LEF (n = 501)	MTX (n = 498)	LEF (n = 1339)
9.2	22.2	10.0	17.0
3.1	12.8	18.1	9.3
3.2	5.8	7.0	4.9
0.4	5.8	16.9	4.9
0.9	9.6	7.8	6.8
7	9.8	4.0	10.3
.9	26.5	24.5	15.1
8	10.8	9.6	9.9
0	16.2	9.8	9.7

or vasculitic diseases with lower doses of steroids.[108] It is uncertain whether it is as effective as other slow-acting anti-rheumatoid drugs in the treatment of active synovitis. It is sometimes prescribed when other drugs are withdrawn due to toxicity or lack of response. GI upset and malaise are relatively common, but haematological dyscrasia and other serious side-effects are uncommon. However, it is associated with an increase in malignant disease in patients on long-term treatment.

Cyclophosphamide

Cyclophosphamide is usually reserved for patients with necrotizing vasculitis. It is effective and has less side-effects, if given as intravenous pulses, often with pulse intravenous methylprednisolone.[47] The initial doses are usually given 1 or 2 weeks apart, but once patients respond to treatment dosage, it is usually continued monthly for 6 months. Blood dyscrasias are common and urinary tract malignancies have been reported. Patients are usually monitored under close hospital supervision.

Tumour necrosis factor (TNF) inhibitors

There are currently two licensed compounds that inhibit TNF and are effective in active RA. Both drugs are extremely expensive, and in many countries this has led to a re-evaluation of healthcare costs for RA. Infliximab is a monoclonal antibody to TNF and is administered as an intravenous infusion: the standard regime is a 3 mg/kg infusion repeated after 2 and 6 weeks, and then every 2 months thereafter (Figure 52).[109] It is only administered in combination with methotrexate. Etanercept is a soluble TNF receptor that is administered twice weekly by subcutaneous injection as monotherapy (Figure 52B).[110] Both compounds have been found to be effective in many patients who were previously resistant to drug therapy, although a significant minority of patients fail to respond. Serious side-effects are uncommon, but there is an increased risk of infection, which may be life threatening. Reactivation of tuberculosis is a particular concern and any evidence of previous tuberculosis is a contraindication to anti-TNF therapy.[111]

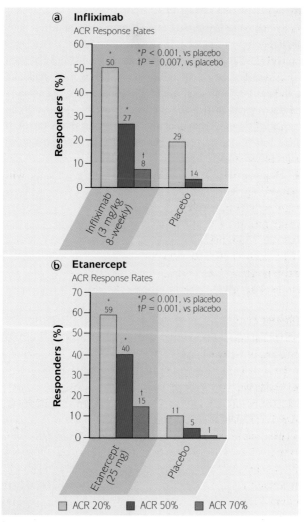

Figure 52. Response rates of TNF inhibitors. Part A reproduced with permission from Moreland LW, Schiff MH, Baumgartner SW *et al. Ann Intern Med* 1999; **130**: 478–486.[110] Part B reproduced with permission from The Lancet (1999; **354**: 1932).[109]

Response to drug therapy

Response to corticosteroids, pulse cyclophosphamide and anti-TNF therapy is rapid, but the response to other DMARDs is usually slow. A response to treatment may sometimes be seen with methotrexate and leflunomide within 4–6 weeks of commencing treatment, but it is unusual to see response to treatment with other drug therapy before 6–8 weeks. Drug response is usually maximal after 4–6 months of treatment. If there is no response after this period, a change in drug treatment is usually considered.

Overview of Other Inflammatory Joint Diseases

Sero-negative spondylo-arthropathies

The sero-negative spondylo-arthropathies (SNSs) are a group of conditions with overlapping features (Table 15). It is often useful to consider the SNSs as a spectrum of a single disease with differing manifestations. Some patients have multiple features, e.g. a patient with Crohn's disease (regional ileitis) and a history of iritis and psoriasis developing ankylosing spondylitis. An enthesitis is a feature in some patients. There is a strong familial link with an association with HLA-B27. It is not unusual to find a complex family history with different manifestations of the SNSs in a number of family members. Undifferentiated spondylo-arthritis refers to patients with some features of this group of diseases, but without sufficient features for any one diagnosis.

Ankylosing spondylitis

Ankylosing spondylitis is the major link between the different manifestations of SNS, as it is associated with all the separate diseases. It is more common in men than women, with a ratio of approximately 5:1, although this may partially reflect under-diagnosis in women. Initial symptoms usually develop from the late teens to early thirties, although the diagnosis may not be made until later in life. Characteristic symptoms are low

Sero-negative spondylo-arthritis
Ankylosing spondylitis
Psoriatic arthritis
Reactive arthritis and Reiter's disease
Enteropathic arthritis
Iritis

Table 15. Sero-negative spondylo-arthritis.

back pain with prolonged early morning stiffness that improves with exercise. Some patients may have diffuse pelvic pain and others may have sciatica. It is typical for symptoms to gradually involve the dorsal and then cervical spine, but the progress of the disease is variable. A minority of patients develop severe disease with unremitting pain, stiffness and restriction in movement. Some patients will develop episodic synovitis in large joints and approximately 5% require hip replacement, although the majority of patients do not have significant disability.

The diagnosis is made on X-ray with bilateral sacroiliitis (Figure 53) and a spinal lesion – either a corner (Romanus) lesion (Figure 54) or a syndesmophyte.[112] Sacroiliitis alone may be seen in any of the SNS conditions. Only 10% of patients develop the appearances of a "bamboo spine" with bridging syndesmophytes at most vertebrae (Figure 55). The acute phase proteins are often raised, but a normal ESR or CRP does not exclude the diagnosis. Although 90% of patients are HLA-B27 positive, this is also found in approximately 7% of Caucasian populations and is only helpful as a guide in borderline cases.

All patients should go swimming regularly and be taught a regime of exercises to be undertaken on a daily basis. There is often a dramatic improvement from NSAIDs, and they should be continued regularly until there is a remission of symptoms. The response to disease-modifying drugs is disappointing.

Psoriatic arthritis

Psoriatic arthritis (PsA) occurs in approximately 5% of patients with psoriasis.[113] Overall, the prognosis is better than RA.[114] The diagnostic criteria are:

(a) a history of psoriasis;

(b) synovitis;

(c) negative rheumatoid factor.

There are five different subsets of disease:[115]

1. Monoarthritis or asymmetric oligoarthritis – the most common presentation of PsA and is usually intermittent.

2. Polyarticular – virtually indistinguishable from RA (see Figure 10).

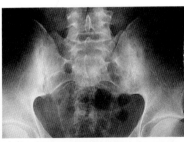

Figure 53. Bilateral sacroiliitis.

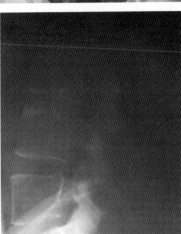

Figure 54. Romanus or corner lesion.

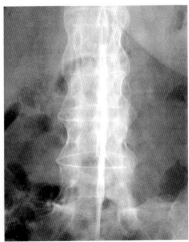

Figure 55. "Bamboo spine".

3. Ankylosing spondylitis.
4. DIP pattern (Figure 56) – peripheral synovitis involving the DIP joints in addition to other joints similar to RA.
5. Arthritis mutilans (Figure 57) – severe destructive arthritis leading to loss of bone and severe deformity.

The management of PsA is similar to that of RA.

Reactive arthritis

Reactive arthritis (ReA) usually presents as a large joint monoarthritis more frequently than a polyarthritis. A dactylitis (sausage finger or toe; Figure 58) is strongly suggestive of ReA or PsA.

Fever, malaise and other systemic symptoms are common. ReA usually follows a viral, GI or urinary infection, including parvovirus, campylobacter, clostridium, salmonella, shigella, yersinia and chlamydial infections. Reiter's disease is a reactive arthritis with urethritis and conjunctivitis; circinate balanitis and keratoderma blenorrhagica (a rash identical to pustular psoriasis; Figure 59) are associated features.[116–118]

The management is similar to acute synovitis from any cause. For persistent disease, either sulphasalazine or methotrexate may be considered.

Enteropathic arthritis

Episodic peripheral synovitis occurs in up to 20% of patients with either ulcerative colitis or Crohn's disease, and reflects the disease activity in the bowel. Ankylosing spondylitis occurs in approximately 7% of patients with inflammatory bowel disease, but spinal disease is largely unrelated to other disease activity. Management is similar to ReA.[119]

Iritis

Iritis or anterior uveitis is associated with all the SNSs and approximately 50% of patients are HLA-B27 positive.[120] Some patients with a history of iritis may develop episodic large joint arthritis and may be diagnosed as undifferentiated SNS. Management is similar to ReA (see Figure 6).

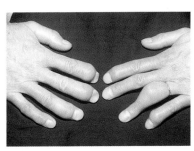

Figure 56. DIP type of psoriatic arthritis.

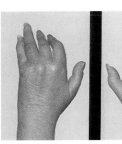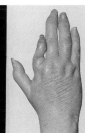

Figure 57. Psoriatic arthritis with arthritis of DIP joints and arthritis mutilans of the index finger.

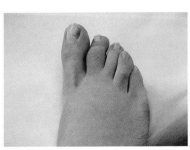

Figure 58. Dactylitis of second toe in psoriatic arthritis.

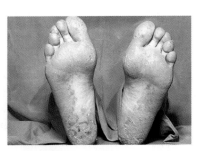

Figure 59. Keratoderma blenorrhagica.

Connective tissue diseases

The connective tissue diseases (CTDs) are a group of auto-immune diseases characterized by antibodies and rheumatic symptoms, often with cutaneous or other systemic features (Table 17). With the exception of RA, they are uncommon in most populations. Although the CTDs are not as close a family as the SNSs, there are several overlap syndromes that may involve any of the diseases and there are some features such as keratoconjunctivitis sicca, nail fold erythema and vasculitis (Figure 60) that are common to all. Some patients do not fulfil any specific criteria for diagnosis and are diagnosed with undifferentiated CTD. Giant cell (cranial or temporal) arteritis is not associated with auto-antibodies but is included for ease of classification (Table 16).

Systemic lupus erythematosus (SLE)[121, 122]

This usually presents in young women with a polyarthralgia. There may be little apparent joint swelling, although some patients have synovitis that is clinically indistinguishable from RA. There may be a history of photosensitivity and mild diffuse

Connective tissue diseases
RA
SLE
Systemic sclerosis
CREST syndrome
Primary Sjögren's
Polymyositis
Dermatomyositis
MCTD
Undifferentiated connective tissue disease
Polyarteritis nodosa
Wegener's granulomatosis
[PMR/giant cell (cranial or temporal) arteritis]

Table 16. Connective tissue diseases.

Auto-antibodies associated with connective tissue diseases	
Antibody	**Clinical interpretation**
ANA	Autoimmune disease chronic infection, drugs, ageing
DNA	SLE, rarely other
Cardiolipin	Recurrent thrombosis and abortion ± SLE
"ENA"	A set of antibodies: see below
Ro (= SSA)	Primary Sjögren's syndrome, SLE, subacute cutaneous LE, congenital heart block
La (= SSB)	As with anti-Ro. In SLE the course is often milder
Sm	SLE, with racial variation
RNP	SLE, mixed connective tissue disease, Raynaud's phenomenon, swollen fingers, myositis
Jo-1, PL-7, PL-12	Myositis and fibrosing alveolitis with Raynaud's, sicca, arthralgias
PM-Scl (= PM1)	Myositis–scleroderma overlap
Ku	SLE, myositis–scleroderma overlap
SL, ribosomal, PCNA, PL-4	Chiefly SLE
XR	Chronic active hepatitis
Centromere (ANA pattern)	CREST syndrome ± primary biliary cirrhosis
Multiple nuclear dots (ANA pattern)	Primary biliary cirrhosis, usually with sicca syndrome
Mitochondria	Primary biliary cirrhosis
cANCA	Wegener's granulomatosis microscopic polyarteritis nodosa
pANCA	Other vasculitides

Table 17. Auto-antibodies associated with connective tissue diseases.

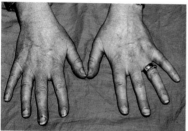

Figure 60. Nail fold erythema with cutaneous vasculitis.

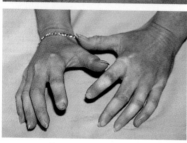

Figure 61. Scleroderma.

alopecia. A butterfly rash is characteristic but is not consistent. Migraine headaches and malaise are common. It is usual to have a positive ANA, but patients with mild lupus may not develop antibodies to dsDNA (Table 18). Renal and cerebral complications are signalled by an increasing titre of dsDNA associated with a fall in C_3. Patients should be managed by an experienced rheumatologist.

Systemic sclerosis (scleroderma)

This is an uncommon disease that usually presents with Raynaud's phenomenon and arthralgia (Figure 61). Dysphagia from oesophageal dysmotility occurs in the majority of patients during the course of the disease, and atonia of the small bowel may lead to bacterial overgrowth and malabsorption. Respiratory complications are common as a result of either inhalational pneumonia or pulmonary fibrosis. Maintaining adequate peripheral circulation is an important aspect of management. There are a number of variants of the condition,[123] including limited cutaneous disease, sometimes termed CREST syndrome because of the presence of *C*alcification, *R*aynaud's, o*E*sophageal dysfunction, *S*clerodactyly and *T*elangiectasia.

Revised criteria of the American Rheumatism Association for the classification of systemic lupus erythematosis

1. Malar rash

2. Discoid rash

3. Photosensitivity

4. Oral ulcers

5. Arthritis

6. Serositis: (a) pleuritis or (b) pericarditis

7. Renal disorder: (a) proteinuria > 0.5 g/24 hours or 3+, persistently, or (b) cellular casts

8. Neurological disorder: (a) seizures or (b) psychosis (having excluded other causes, e.g. drugs)

9. Haematological disorder: (a) haemolytic anaemia, (b) leucopenia of <4.0 $\times$ 10^9/l on two or more occasions, (c) lymphopenia of <1.5 $\times$ 10^9/l on two or more occasions, (d) thrombocytopenia <100 $\times$ 10^9/l

10. Immunological disorders: (a) positive LE cell, (b) raised anti-native DNA antibody binding, (c) anti-Sm antibody or (d) false-positive serological test for syphilis, present for at least 6 months

11. Antinuclear antibody in raised titre: "… A person shall be said to have SLE if four or more of the 11 criteria are present, serially or simultaneously, during any interval of observation"

Table 18. Revised criteria of the American Rheumatism Association for the classification of systemic lupus erythematosus.

Primary Sjögren's syndrome

This should be considered particularly in middle aged women with keratoconjunctivitis sicca and arthralgia. A positive Ro or La antibody confirms the diagnosis.[124] Management is usually symptomatic unless there are associated systemic features.

Polymyositis/dermatomyositis

These are rare conditions presenting with myalgia and muscle weakness. The rash of dermatomyositis is an erythematous violaceous eruption typically occurring in a peri-orbital distribution and on the extensor surfaces of the MCP and PIP joints. There is an association with malignancy in elderly patients. Muscle enzymes are almost invariably elevated and the diagnosis is confirmed with EMG and muscle biopsy.[125]

Polyarteritis nodosa

Polyarteritis nodosa (PAN) is an uncommon condition that typically presents in middle-aged or elderly men with myalgia, weight loss and night sweats. Some patients have a frank arthritis suggestive of RA, but the development of abdominal pain, hypertension or neurological complications, including mononeuritis multiplex, are virtually diagnostic. Some patients may present with acute or sub-acute renal failure. Antibodies to neutrophil cytoplasmic antigens[126] are associated with certain forms of PAN, but are found in most patients with Wegener's granulomatosis, a condition with similar features to PAN but characterized by respiratory tract granulomata. Treatment of both diseases is with steroids and cyclophosphamide.

Future Developments

The concept of targeted therapies for arthritis is the beginning of a new approach to treatment. The COX-2 inhibitors were among the first designer drugs – identifying part of a pathological process and developing a drug for a specific action. Emerging data on the role of COX-2 in the CNS[127] may lead to the development of more effective compounds that are directed to specific sites integral to the mediation of pain.

The introduction of the first biological therapies for arthritis, against TNFα, is the start of a revolution in the treatment of inflammatory diseases. Greater understanding of the mechanisms of inflammation has led to new applications being considered, not only for these compounds, but also for a range of other "biologics" in development. Monoclonal antibodies can be developed against specific targets that are integral to the inflammatory cascade, although the concerns about the potential toxicity of interfering with fundamental physiological processes are real. However, for the first time we can contemplate in the future the possibility of a cure for RA.

The current treatment of OA is unsatisfactory: there is no treatment that will arrest the progression of cartilage destruction and it is doubtful whether a biological target will be identified that will stop cartilage degradation. However, with the increased understanding of the genetic factors in OA, and with the introduction of targeted gene therapy for some conditions, it is possible to consider that this therapy may be a future option for the treatment of some patients with OA.

In tandem with these exciting scientific developments are difficult questions about funding in healthcare. Biological treatment is considerably more costly to develop and manufacture than traditional therapies, and whether resources will be available to meet the demand is a concern.

Frequently Asked Questions

Are there any diets that help?

Only for weight reduction and a low purine diet in gout (avoid offal, large quantities of red meat and certain small fish, e.g. anchovies). Diets for RA are usually unhelpful. There is a small theoretical benefit from consumption of large amount of oily fish, but this is not only impractical but is unlikely to have any significant effect on outcome.

Does the weather affect arthritis?

Wet weather increases the symptoms, probably because the atmospheric pressure is low, resulting in a relative increase in joint pressure.

Are cod liver oil and glucosamine effective?

Cod liver oil is a good source of vitamin D, but is unlikely to have an effect on rheumatic symptoms. The data on glucosamine are interesting. There are a number of small studies that found a small analgesic effect and one study found a retardation in progression of OA of the knee. This observation needs confirmation. Its mode of action is unclear.

Is there a limit to the number of joint injections?

This is largely dictated by common sense. If a number of injections do not have prolonged benefit, then it is preferable to consider other treatment. There are some laboratory data to suggest that there may be a negative effect on cartilage from repeated injections, but this is balanced by the benefit of reducing the detrimental effect of inflammation. However, as a general guide do not repeat an intra-articular injection more than three or four times in one year.

References

1. Linaker CH, Walker-Bone K, Palmer K, Cooper C. Frequency of regional musculoskeletal disorders. *Baillieres Clin Rheumatol* 1999; **13**:197–215.

2. van Saase JL, van Romunde LK, Cats A *et al*. Epidemiology of OA: Zoetermeer survey. Comparison of radiological osteoarthritis in a Dutch population with that in 10 other populations. *Ann Rheum Dis* 1989; **48**: 271.

3. Spector TD. Rheumatoid arthritis. *Rheum Dis Clin North Am* 1990; **16**: 513.

4. Lawrence RC, Helmick CG, Arnett FC *et al*. Estimates of the prevalence of arthritis and selected musculoskeletal disorders in the United States. *Arthritis Rheum* 1998; **41**: 778.

5. Parke AL, Wilson D, Maier D. The prevalence of antiphospholipid antibodies in women with recurrent spontaneous abortion, women with successful pregnancies, and women who have never been pregnant. *Arth Rheum* 1991; **34**:1231.

6. Martinez-Borra J, Gonzalez S, Lopez-Larrea C. Genetic factors predisposing to spondyloarthropathies. *Arth Rheum* 2000; **43**: 485.

7. Solomon L. Clinical features of osteoarthritis. In: Kelley WN, Hams ED Jr, Ruddy S, Sledge CB, editors. *Textbook of Rheumatology*. Philadelphia: W.B. Saunders, 1996, p. 1383.

8. Cammarata RJ, Rodnan GP, Fennell RH. Serum anti-gammaglobulin and antinuclear factors in the aged. *J Am Med Assoc* 1967; **199**: 455.

9. Felson DT, Zhang YO, Anthony JM *et al*. Weight loss reduces the risk for symptomatic knee osteoarthritis in women: the Framingham study. *Ann Intern Med* 1992; **116**: 535.

10. Hayes J, McKenna F. Sleeping in a soft collar is effective treatment for the symptoms of cervical spondylosis. *Ann Rheum Dis* 2002; 61(Supp 1): 488.

11. Green J, McKenna F, Redfern EJ, Chamberlain MA. Home exercises are as effective as out-patient hydrotherapy for osteoarthritis of the hip. *Br J Rheumatol* 1993; **32**: 812–815.

12. Chamberlain MA, Care G, Harfield B. Physiotherapy in osteoarthrosis of the knees. A controlled trial of hospital versus home exercises. *Int Rehab Med* 1982; **4**: 101–106.

13. Pickavance L, Griffiths G, McKenna F. Diclofenac is a better analgesic than paracetamol in patients with osteoarthritis of the hip, knee and lumbar spine. *Br J Rheumatol* 1995; **34**(Suppl 1): 37.

14. Pincus T, Koch GG, Sokka T *et al*. A randomized, double-blind, crossover clinical trial of diclofenac plus misoprostol versus acetaminophen in patients with osteoarthritis of the hip or knee. *Arth Rheum* 2000; **44**: 1587–1598.

15. Larkai EN, Smith JL, Lidsky MD, Graham DY. Gastroduodenal mucosa and dyspeptic symptoms in arthritic patients during chronic nonsteroidal anti-inflammatory drug use. *Am J Gastroenterol* 1987; **82**: 1153.

16. Mason J, McKenna F. Gastric ulceration from NSAIDs does not cause dyspepsia. *Ann Rheum Dis* 2002; 61 (Suppl 1): 42.

17. Simon LS, Hatoum TH, Bittman RM *et al*. Risk factors for serious nonsteroidal-induced gastrointestinal complications: regression analysis of the MUCOSA trial. *Fam Med* 1996; **28**: 202.

18. Griffin MR, Piper JM, Daugherty JR *et al*. Nonsteroidal antiinflammatory drug use and increased risk for peptic ulcer disease in elderly persons. *Ann Intern Med* 1991; **114**: 257.

19. Gabriel SE, Jaaklimainen L, Bombadier C. Risk for serious gastrointestinal complications related to use of nonsteroidal antiinflammatory drugs: a meta-analysis. *Ann Intern Med* 1991; **115**: 787.

20. Singh G, Triadafilopoulos G. Epidemiology of NSAID induced gastrointestinal complications. *J Rheumatol* 1999; **26**(Suppl 56): 18–24.

21. Graham DY, Agrawal NM, Roth SH. Prevention of NSAID-induced gastric ulcer with misoprostol: multicentre, double-blind, placebo-controlled trial. *Lancet* 1988; **2**: 1277.

22. Silverstein FE, Graham DY, Senior JR *et al*. Misoprostol reduces serious gastrointestinal complications in patients with rheumatoid arthritis receiving nonsteroidal anti-inflammatory drugs. *Ann Intern Med* 1995; **123**: 214.

23. McKenna F. Diclofenac/misoprostol: the European clinical experience. *J Rheumatol* 1998; **25**(551): 21–30.

24. Ehsanullah RS, Page MC, Tildesley G, Wood JR. Prevention of gastroduodenal damage induced by non-steroidal anti-inflammatory drugs: controlled trial of ranitidine. *Br Med J* 1988; **297**: 1017.

25. Robinson MG, Griffin JW Jr, Bowers J *et al*. Effect of ranitidine on gastroduodenal damage induced by nonsteroidal anti-inflammatory drugs. *Dig Dis Sci* 1989; **34**: 424.

26. Graham DY. High-dose famotidine for prevention of NSAID ulcers? *Gastroenterology* 1997; **112**: 2143.

27. Hawkey CJ, Karrasch JA, Szczepanski L *et al*. Omeprazole compared with misoprostol for ulcers associated with nonsteroidal antiinflammatory drugs. *New Engl J Med* 1998; **338**:727.

28. Oddsson E, Gudjonsson H, Thjodleifsson B. Protective effect of omeprazole or ranitidine against naproxen induced damage to the human gastroduodenal mucosa. *Scand J Gastroenterol* 1990; **13**(Suppl 176): 25.

29. Vane JR. Inhibition of prostaglandin synthesis as a mechanism of action for the aspirin-like drugs. *Nature* 1971; **231**: 232.

30. McKenna F. Cox-2: separating myth from reality. *Scand J Rheumatol* 1999; **28**(Suppl 109): 19–29.

31. Soll AH. NSAIDS and peptic ulcer disease. *Ann Intern Med* 1991; **114**: 307–319.

32. Quigley EM *et al*. pH of the microclimate lining gastric and duodenal mucosa in vivo. *Gastroenterology* 1987; **92**: 1876–1884.

33. Simon LS, Weaver AL, Graham DY *et al*. Anti-inflammatory and upper gastrointestinal effects of celecoxib in rheumatoid arthritis: a randomized controlled trial. *J Am Med Assoc* 1999; **282**: 1921.

34. Laine L, Harper S, Simon T *et al*. A randomized trial comparing the effect of rofecoxib, a cyclooxygenase 2-specific inhibitor, with that of ibuprofen on the gastroduodenal mucosa of patients with osteoarthritis. *Gastroenterology* 1999; **117**: 776.

35. Emery P, Zeidler H, Kvien TK *et al*. Celecoxib versus diclofenac in long-term management of rheumatoid arthritis: randomised double-blind comparison. *Lancet* 1999; **354**: 2106.

36. McKenna F, Borenstein D, Wendt H, Wallemark C, Lefkowith J, Geis GS. Celecoxib versus diclofenac in the management of osteoarthritis of the knee – a placebo-controlled, randomised double-blind comparison. *Scand J Rheum* 2001; **30**: 11–18.

37. McKenna F, Arguelles L, Burke T, Lefkowith J, Geis GS. Upper gastrointestinal tolerability of celecoxib compared with diclofenac in the treatment of osteoarthritis and rheumatoid arthritis. *Clin Exp Rheumatol* 2002; **20**: 35–43.

38. Day R, Morrison B, Luza A *et al*. A randomized trial of the efficacy and tolerability of the COX-2 inhibitor rofecoxib vs ibuprofen in patients with osteoarthritis. *Arch Intern Med* 2000; **160**: 1781.

39. Hawkey C, Laine L, Simon T *et al*. Comparison of the effect of rofecoxib (a cyclooxygenase 2 inhibitor), ibuprofen, and placebo on the gastroduodenal mucosa of patients with osteoarthritis. *Arth Rheum* 2000; **43**: 370.

40. Silverstein FE, Faich G, Goldstein JL *et al*. Gastrointestinal toxicity with celecoxib vs nonsteroidal anti-inflammatory drugs for osteoarthritis and rheumatoid arthritis. The CLASS study: a randomized controlled trial. *J Am Med Assoc* 2000; **284**: 1247.

41. Bombardier C, Laine L, Reicin A *et al*. Comparison of upper gastrointestinal toxicity of rofecoxib and naproxen in patients with rheumatoid arthritis. VIGOR Study Group. *New Engl J Med* 2000; **343**: 1520.

42. Harris RC. Cyclooxygenase-2 in the kidney. *J Am Soc Nephrol* 24300; **11**: 2387–2394.

43. Van Hecken A, Schwartz JI, Depre M *et al*. Comparative inhibitory activity of rofecoxib, meloxicam, diclofenac, ibuprofen, and naproxen on COX-2 versus COX-1 in healthy volunteers. *J Clin Pharmacol* 2000; **40**: 1109.

44. Corkill MM, Kirkham BW, Chikanza IC *et al*. Intramuscular depot methylprednisolone induction of chrysotherapy in rheumatoid arthritis: a 24 week randomized controlled trial. *Br J Rheumatol* 1990; **29**: 274.

45. Choy ES, Kingsley GH, Corkill MM, Panayi GS. Intramuscular methylprednisolone is superior to pulse oral methylprednisolone during the induction phase of chrysotherapy. *Br J Rheumatol* 1993; **32**: 734.

46. Radia M, Furst DE. Comparison of three pulse methylprednisolone regimens in the treatment of rheumatoid arthritis. *J Rheumatol* 1988; **15**: 242.

47. Scott DG, Bacon PA. Intravenous cyclophosphamide plus methylprednisolone in the treatment of systemic rheumatoid vasculitis. *Am J Med* 1984; **76**: 377.

48. Pilowsky I, Hallett EC, Bassett DL *et al*. A controlled study of amitriptyline in the treatment of chronic pain. *Pain* 1982; **14**: 169.

49. Godfrey RG. A guide to the understanding and use of tricycle antidepressants in the overall management of fibromyalgia and other chronic pain syndromes. *Arch Intern Med* 1996; **156**: 1047.

50. Swerdlow M. Review: Anticonvulsant drugs and chronic pain. *Clin Neuropharmacol* 1984; **7**: 51.

51. McKenna F, Hume K. Abnormalities of sleep EEG in fibromyalgia. *Ann Rheum Dis* 2002; **61** (Suppl 1): 454.

52. Wolfe F, Ross K, Anderson J, Russell IJ *et al*. The prevalence and characteristics of fibromyalgia in the general population. *Arth Rheum* 1995; **38**: 19.

53. Jaeschke R, Adachi J, Guyatt G *et al*. Clinical usefulness of amitriptyline in fibromyalgia: the results of 23 N-of-1 randomized controlled trials. *J Rheumatol* 1991; **18**: 447-451..

54. Wolfe F, Smythe HA, Yunus MB *et al*. The American College of Rheumatology 1990 criteria for the classification of fibromyalgia: report of the Multicenter Criteria Committee. *Arth Rheum* 1990; **33**: 160.

55. Harrington JM, Carter JT, Birrell L, Gompertz D. Surveillance case definitions for work related upper limb pain syndromes. *Occup Environ Med* 1998; **55**: 1264–1271.

56. Cicuttini FM, Spector TD. Genetics of osteoarthritis. *Ann Rheum Dis* 1996; **55**: 665.

57. Spector TD, Cicuttini F, Baker J *et al*. Genetic influences on osteoarthritis in women: a twin study. *Br Med J* 1996; **312**: 940.

58. van Saase JL, van Romunde LK, Cats A *et al*. Epidemiology of osteoarthritis: Zoetermeer survey. Comparison of radiological osteoarthritis in a Dutch population with that in 10 other populations. *Ann Rheum Dis* 1989; **48**: 271.

59. Cooper C, Egger P, Coggon D *et al*. Generalized osteoarthritis in women: pattern of joint involvement and approaches to definition for epidemiological studies. *J Rheumatol* 1996; **23**: 1938.

60. Oliveria SA, Felson DT, Klein RA *et al*. Estrogen replacement therapy and the development of osteoarthritis. *Epidemiology* 1996; **7**: 415.

61. Nevitt MC, Lane NE, Scott JC *et al*. Radiographic osteoarthritis of the hip and bone mineral density. *Arth Rheum* 1995; **38**: 907.

62. Hart DJ, Mootoosamy I, Doyle DV, Spector TD. The relationship between osteoarthritis and osteoporosis in the general population: the Chingford Study. *Ann Rheum Dis* 1994; **53**: 158.

63. Hart DJ, Spector TD. The relationship of obesity, fat distribution and osteoarthritis in women in the general population: the Chingford study. *J Rheumatol* 1993; **20**: 331.

64. Felson DT, Zhang YO, Anthony JM *et al*. Weight loss reduces the risk for symptomatic knee osteoarthritis in women: the Framingham study. *Ann Intern Med* 1992; **116**: 535.

65. Hartz AJ, Fischer ME, Bril G *et al*. The association of obesity with joint pain and osteoarthritis in the HANES data. *J Chronic Dis* 1986; **39**: 311.

66. Gelber AC, Hochberg MC, Mead LA *et al*. Body mass index in young men and the risk of subsequent knee and hip osteoarthritis. *Am J Med* 1999; **107**: 542.

67. Chakravarty K, Pharoah PD, Scott DGI. A randomized controlled study of post-injection rest following intra-articular steroid therapy for knee synovitis. *Br J Rheumatol* 1994; **33**: 464.

68. Hochberg MC. Prognosis of osteoarthritis. *Ann Rheum Dis* 1996; **55**: 685.

69. Brooks RC, McGee SR. Diagnostic dilemmas in polymyalgia rheumatica. *Arch Intern Med* 1997; **157**: 1162–1168.

70. Salvarani C, Cantini F, Olivieri I, Hunder GS. Polymyalgia rheumatica: a disorder of extraarticular synovial structures? *J Rheumatol* 1999; **26**: 517.

71. Myklebust G, Gran JT. A prospective study of 287 patients with polymyalgia rheumatic and temporal arteritis: clinical and laboratory manifestations at onset of disease and at the time of diagnosis. *Br J Rheumatol* 1996; **35**: 1161.

72. Chuang TY, Hunder GG, Ilstrup DM *et al*. Polymyalgia rheumatica. A 10-year epidemiologic and clinical study. *Ann Intern Med* 1982; **97**: 672.

73. Cantini F, Salvarani C, Olivieri I *et al*. Erythrocyte sedimentation rate and C-reactive protein in the evaluation of disease activity and severity in polymyalgia rheumatica: a prospective follow-up study. *Semin Arth Rheum* 2000; **30**: 17–24.

74. Nichols T, Nugent CA, Tyler FH. Diurnal variation in suppression of adrenal function by glucocorticoids. *J Clin Endocrinol Metab* 1965; **25**: 343.

75. Fauci AS. Alternate-day corticosteroid therapy. *Am J Med* 1978; **64**: 729–731.

76. Terkeltaub RA. Pathogenesis and treatment of crystal-induced inflammation. In: Koopman WJ, editor. *Arthritis and Allied Conditions: A Textbook of Rheumatology*, 13th Edition. Baltimore: Williams & Wilkins, 1997; p. 2085.

77. Macfarlane DG, Dieppe PA. Diuretic-induced gout in elderly women. *Br J Rheumatol* 1985; **24**: 155.

78. Grahame R. Scott JT. Clinical survey of 354 patients with gout. *Ann Rheum Dis* 1970; **29**: 461–468.

79. Kahn AM. Effect of diuretics on the renal handling of urate. *Semin Nephrol* 1988; **8**: 305–314.

80. Rundles RW. The development of allopurinol. *Arch Intern Med* 1985; **145**: 1492–1503.

81. Wallace SL, Singer JZ. Therapy in gout. *Rheum Dis Clin North Am* 1988; **14**: 441–457.

82. Kunkl RW, Duncan G, Watson D. Colchicine myopathy and neuropathy. *New Engl J Med* 1987; **316**: 1562–1568.

83. Ryan LM, McCarty DJ. Calcium pyrophosphate crystal deposition disease, pseudogout, and articular chondrocalcinosis. In: Koopman WJ, editor. *Arthritis and Allied Conditions*, 13th Edition. Baltimore: Williams & Wilkins, 1997; pp. 2103–2125.

84. Spector TD. Rheumatoid arthritis. *Rheum Dis Clin North Am* 1990; **16**: 513.

85. Fleming A, Crown JM, Corbett M. Early rheumatoid disease. I. Onset. II. Patterns of joint involvement. *Ann Rheum Dis* 1976; **35**: 357.

86. Pincus T, Callahan LF. Reassessment of twelve traditional paradigms concerning the diagnosis, prevalence, morbidity and mortality of rheumatoid arthritis. *Scand J Rheumatol* 1989; **79**(Suppl): 67–96.

87. McKenna F, Wright V. Pain in rheumatoid arthritis. *Ann Rheum Dis* 1985; **44**: 805.

88. McKenna F, Wright V. Clinical manifestations of rheumatoid arthritis. In: Utsinger PD, Zvaifler NJ, Ehrlich GE, editors. *Rheumatoid Arthritis*. Philadelphia: J.P. Lippincott, 1985.

89. Jacoby RK, Jayson MIV, Cosh JA. Onset, early stages and prognosis of rheumatoid arthritis: a clinical study of 100 patients with 11 year follow-up. *Br Med J* 1973; **2**: 96.

90. Lehtinen JT, Kaarela K, Belt EA *et al*. Incidence of acromioclavicular joint involvement in rheumatoid arthritis: a 15 year endpoint study. *J Rheumatol* 1999; **26**: 1239.

91. Wolfe F, Sharp JT. Radiographic outcome of recent onset rheumatoid arthritis. *Arth Rheum* 1998; **41**: 1571.

92. McKenna F. Clinical and laboratory assessments of outcome in rheumatoid arthritis. *Br J Rheumatol* 1988; **27**(Suppl): 55–60.

93. Chamberlain MA, Corbett M. Carpal tunnel syndrome in early rheumatoid arthritis. *Ann Rheum Dis* 1970; **29**: 149.

94. Pincus T, Marcum SB, Callahan LF. Longterm drug therapy for rheumatoid arthritis in seven rheumatology private practices: II. Second line drugs and prednisone. *J Rheumatol* 1992; **19**(12): 1885–1894.

95. Levy GD, Munz SJ, Paschal J *et al*. Incidence of hydroxychloroquine retinopathy in 1207 patients in a large multicenter outpatient practice. *Arth Rheum* 1997; **40**: 1482.

96. Antimalarial workshop. *J Rheumatol* 1997; **24**: 1393.

97. Bienfang D, Coblyn JS, Liang MH, Corzillius M. Hydroxychloroquine retinopathy despite regular ophthalmologic evaluation: a consecutive series. *J Rheumatol* 2000; **27**: 2703.

98. Box SA, Pullar T. Sulphasalazine in the treatment of rheumatoid arthritis. *Br J Rheumatol* 1997; **36**: 382–386.

99. Weinblatt M, Kaplan H, Germain BF *et al*. Methotrexate in rheumatoid arthritis: a five year prospective multicenter study. *Arth Rheum* 1994; **37**: 1492.

100. Kremer JM. Safety, efficacy, and mortality in a long-term cohort of patients with rheumatoid arthritis taking methotrexate: follow-up after a mean of 13.3 years. *Arth Rheum* 1997; **40**: 984.

101. Barrera P, Laan RFJM, van Riel PLCM *et al*. Methotrexate-related pulmonary complications in rheumatoid arthritis. *Ann Rheum Dis* 1994; **53**: 434.

102. Prakash A, Jarvis B. Leflunomide: a review of its use in active rheumatoid arthritis. *Drugs* 1999; **58**: 1137.

103. Smolen JS *et al*. Efficacy and safety of leflunomide compared with placebo and SAS in active RA. *Lancet* 1999; **353**: 259.

104. Strand V *et al*. Treatment of active RA with leflunomide compared with placebo and MTX. *Arch Intern Med* 1999; **159**: 2542.

105. Emery P. A comparison of the efficacy and safety of leflunomide and MTX for the treatment of RA. *Rheumatology* 2000; **39**: 655.

106. van Jaarsveld CH, Jahangier ZN, Jacobs JW *et al*. Toxicity of anti-rheumatic drugs in a randomized clinical trial of early rheumatoid arthritis. *Rheumatology (Oxford)* 2000; **39**: 1374–1382.

107. Gordon DA. Gold compounds and penicillamine in rheumatic diseases. In: Kelley WN, Harris ED, Ruddy S, Sledge CB, editors. *Textbook of Rheumatology*, 5th Edition, Chap. 48. Philadelphia: W.B. Saunders, 1997; pp. 759–769.

108. Leib ES, Restivo C, Paulus HU. Immunosuppressive and corticosteroid therapy of polyarteritis nodosa. *Am J Med* 1979; **67**: 941.

109. Maini R, St Clair EW, Breedveld F *et al*. Infliximab (chimeric anti-tumour necrosis factor alpha monoclonal antibody) versus placebo in rheumatoid arthritis patients receiving concomitant methotrexate: a randomized phase III trial. *Lancet* 1999; **354**: 1932.

110. Moreland LW, Schiff MH, Baumgartner SW *et al*. Etanercept therapy in rheumatoid arthritis. A randomized, controlled trial. *Ann Intern Med* 1999; **130**: 478–486.

111. Furst DE, Breedveld FC, Burmester GR *et al*. Updated consensus statement on tumour necrosis factor blocking agents for the treatment of rheumatoid arthritis. *Ann Rheum Dis* 2000; **59**(Suppl 1): i1–2.

112. Calin A, MacKay K, Santos H, Brophy S. A new dimension to outcome: application of the Bath Ankylosing Spondylitis Radiology Index. *J Rheumatol* 1999; **26**: 988.

113. Shbeeb M, Uramoto KM, Gibson LE *et al*. The epidemiology of psoriatic arthritis in Olmsted County, Minnesota, USA, 1982–1991. *J Rheumatol* 2000; **27**: 1247.

114. Jones SM, Armas JB, Cohen MG *et al*. Psoriatic arthritis: outcome of disease subsets and relationship of joint disease to nail and skin disease. *Br J Rheumatol* 1994; **33**: 834.

115. Wright V, Moll JMH. Psoriatic arthritis. *Bull Rheum Dis* 1971; **21**: 627.

116. Yu DT, Thompson GT. Clinical, epidemiological and pathogenesis of reactive arthritis. *Food Microbiol* 1994; **11**: 97.

117. Hughes RA, Keat AC. Reiter's syndrome and reactive arthritis: a current view. *Semin Arth Rheum* 1994; **24**: 190.

118. Kvien T, Glennas A, Melby K *et al*. Reactive arthritis: incidence, triggering agent and clinical presentation. *J Rheumatol* 1994; **21**: 115.

119. McKenna F, Wright V. Arthritic manifestations of inflammatory bowel disease. *Int Med Spec* 1987; **8**: 163–171.

120. Rosenbaum JT. Acute anterior uveitis and spondyloarthropathies. *Rheum Dis Clin North Am* 1992; **18**: 143–151.

121. Boumpas DT, Austin HA III, Fessler BJ *et al*. Systemic lupus erythematosus: emerging concepts. Part 1: Renal, neuropsychiatric, cardiovascular, pulmonary, and hematologic disease. *Ann Intern Med* 1995; **122**: 940–950.

122. Boumpas DT, Fessler BJ, Austin HA III *et al*. Systemic lupus erythematosus: emerging concepts. Part 2: Dermatologic and joint disease, the antiphospholipid antibody syndrome, pregnancy and hormonal therapy, morbidity and mortality and pathogenesis. *Ann Intern Med* 1995; **123**: 42–53.

123. Black CM. Scleroderma – clinical aspects. *J Intern Med* 1993; **234**: 115–118.

124. Hanley JB, Alexander EL, Bias WB *et al*. Anti-Ro (SSA) and anti-La (SSB) in patients with Sjögren's syndrome. *Arth Rheum* 1986; **29**: 196–206.

125. Bohan A, Peter JB, Bowman RL, Pearson CM. Computer-assisted analysis of 153 patients with polymyositis and dermatomyositis. *Medicine (Baltimore)* 1977; **56**: 255–286.

126. Hoffman GS, Specks U. Antineutrophil cytoplasmic antibodies. *Arth Rheum* 1998; **41**: 1521–1537.

127. Samad TA, Moore KA, Sapirstein A *et al*. Interleukin-1b-mediated induction of Cox-2 in the CNS contributes to inflammatory pain hypersensitivity. *Nature* 2001; **410**: 471–475.

Appendix 1 – Drugs

Non-steroidal anti-inflammatory agents (NSAIDs)

Drug	Format	Trade name	Preparation	Strength	Doses used in arthritis (adult)	Comments	Side effects
Non-steroidal anti-inflammatory agents (NSAIDs) Aceclofenac	Oral	Preservex	Tablet	100mg	100mg 2 times/d	Take with or after food	Gastrointestinal discomfort, nausea, diarrhoea; gastrointestinal bleeding and ulceration; hypersensitivity reactions; headache, dizziness, vertigo, hearing disturbances
Acemetacin	Oral	Emflex	Capsule	60mg	60mg 2–3 times/d	Glycolic acid ester of indometacin; take with or after food	Gastrointestinal discomfort, nausea, diarrhoea; gastrointestinal bleeding and ulceration; hypersensitivity reactions; headache, dizziness, vertigo, hearing disturbances
Azapropazone	Oral	Rheumox	Capsule Tablet	300mg 600mg	300–600mg 2–4 times/d (max. 1.2g/d); elderly max. 300mg 2 times/d	Use restricted to rheumatoid arthritis when other NSAIDs have failed; avoid direct exposure to sunlight or use sunblock; take with or after food	Gastrointestinal discomfort, nausea, diarrhoea; gastrointestinal bleeding and ulceration (may be severe); hypersensitivity reactions (may be severe); headache, dizziness, vertigo, hearing disturbances; photosensitivity reactions

Non-steroidal anti-inflammatory agents (NSAIDs) (continued)

Drug	Format	Trade name	Preparation	Strength	Doses used in arthritis (adult)	Comments	Side effects
Dexketoprofen	Oral	Keral	Tablet	25mg	12.5-25mg 3-4 times daily (max. 75mg/d); elderly max. 50mg/d	Isomer of ketoprofen; used for short term treatment of pain; take with or after food	Gastrointestinal discomfort, nausea, diarrhoea; gastrointestinal bleeding and ulceration; hypersensitivity reactions; headache, dizziness, vertigo, hearing disturbances
				75mg			
Diclofenac sodium	Oral	Diclomax SR	M/R capsule	75mg	75-150mg 1-2 times/d (max. 150mg)	Take with or after food	Gastrointestinal discomfort, nausea, diarrhoea; gastrointestinal bleeding and ulceration; hypersensitivity reactions; headache, dizziness, vertigo, hearing disturbances
		Diclomax Retard	M/R capsule	100mg	100mg/d		
		Motifene	M/R E/C capsule	25mg, 50mg	75mg 1-2 times/d		
		Voltarol	Tablet	75mg	75-150mg/d		
		Voltarol SR	M/R tablet	100mg	75mg 1-2 times/d		
		Voltarol Retard	M/R tablet		100mg/d		
		Voltarin	Tablet	50, 75mg	150-200mg/d		
		Cetaflau	Tablet	100mg	100-200mg/d		

Non-steroidal anti-inflammatory agents (NSAIDs) (continued)

Drug	Format	Trade name	Preparation	Strength	Doses used in arthritis (adult)	Comments	Side effects
		Arthrotec	Tablet	50mg, 75mg (twice daily) (with misoprostol 200mcg)	1 tablet 2-3 times/d	Used as prophylaxis against NSAID-induced gastroduodenal ulceration; contraindicated in pregnant women and women planning a pregnancy	
	Topical	Voltarol	Emulgel	1%	Apply 3-4 times/d		Hypersensitivity reactions
	Rectal	Voltarol	Suppository	12.5mg, 25mg, 50mg, 100mg	75-100mg/d in divided doses		Rectal irritation and occasional bleeding
Diflunisal	Oral	Dolobid	Tablet	250mg, 500mg	500-1000mg 1-2 times/d (max. 1000mg)	Take with or after food	Gastrointestinal discomfort, nausea, diarrhoea; gastrointestinal bleeding and ulceration; hypersensitivity reactions; headache, dizziness, vertigo, hearing disturbances
Etodolac	Oral	Lodine SR	M/R tablet	600mg	600mg/d	Take with or after food	Gastrointestinal discomfort, nausea, diarrhoea; gastrointestinal bleeding and ulceration; hypersensitivity reactions; headache, dizziness, vertigo, hearing disturbances

Non-steroidal anti-inflammatory agents (NSAIDs) (continued)

Drug	Format	Trade name	Preparation	Strength	Doses used in arthritis (adult)	Comments	Side effects
		Lodine	Tablet	800mg	800mg/d		Use with caution in people with impaired renal and hepatic function, heart failure, those on diuretics and older patients.
Felbinac	Topical	Traxam	Foam, gel	3%	Apply 2–4 times/d		Hypersensitivity reactions
Fenbufen	Oral	Lederfen	Capsule	300mg	300mg mane/600mg nocte	Active metabolite of fenbufen	Gastrointestinal discomfort, nausea, diarrhoea; gastrointestinal bleeding and ulceration; hypersensitivity reactions (high risk); headache, dizziness, vertigo, hearing disturbances; erythema multiforme; Stevens-Johnson syndrome
			Tablet	300mg, 450mg	450mg 2 times/d	Take with or after food	
Fenoprofen	Oral	Fenopron	Tablet	300mg, 600mg	300–600mg 3-4 times/d (max. 3g/d)	Take with or after food	Gastrointestinal discomfort, nausea, diarrhoea; gastrointestinal bleeding and ulceration; hypersensitivity reactions; headache, dizziness, vertigo, hearing disturbances
		Nalfon	Tablet	300mg, 600mg	1.2–2.4g/24h		
Flurbiprofen	Oral	Froben	Tablet	50mg, 100mg, 200mg	150–200mg/d in divided doses	Take with or after food	Gastrointestinal discomfort, nausea, diarrhoea; gastrointestinal bleeding and ulceration; hypersensitivity reactions; headache, dizziness, vertigo, hearing disturbances
		Froben SR	Capsule		200mg/d		
		Ansaid	Tablet	100mg	100–200mg/d		
	Rectal	Froben	Suppository	100mg	100–200mg/d in divided doses		Rectal irritation and occasional bleeding

Non-steroidal anti-inflammatory agents (NSAIDs) (continued)

Drug	Format	Trade name	Preparation	Strength	Doses used in arthritis (adult)	Comments	Side effects
Ibuprofen	Oral	Brufen	Tablet	200mg, 400mg, 600mg	1200-1800mg in 3-4 divided doses (max. 2400mg/d)	Take with or after food	Gastrointestinal discomfort, nausea, diarrhoea; gastrointestinal bleeding and ulceration; hypersensitivity reactions; headache, dizziness, vertigo, hearing disturbances
		Brufen	Syrup	100mg/5ml	1200-1800mg in 3-4 divided doses (max. 2400mg/d)		
		Brufen Retard	M/R tablet	800mg	1600mg/d		
		Fenbid	Spansule	300mg	300-900mg 2 times/d		
		Codafen Contiuus	M/R tablet	300mg (with codeine 20mg)	1-2 tablets 2 times/d		
		Motrin	Tablet	200, 400, 600, 800mg	1200-3200mg/d		
	Topical	Ibugel	Gel	5%, 10%	Apply 3-4 times/d		Hypersensitivity reactions
Indometacin	Oral	Indocid	Capsule	25mg, 50mg	50-200mg/d in divided doses	Caution patients about dizziness if driving; take with or after food	Gastrointestinal discomfort, nausea, diarrhoea (frequent); gastrointestinal bleeding and ulceration; hypersensitivity

Non-steroidal anti-inflammatory agents (NSAIDs) (continued)

Drug	Format	Trade name	Preparation	Strength	Doses used in arthritis (adult)	Comments	Side effects
		Indocid R Flexinl	M/R capsule M/R tablet	75mg 25mg, 50mg,	75mg 1-2 times/d 25-200mg/d in divided doses		reactions; headache, dizziness and light-headedness, vertigo, hearing disturbances
		Indocin		75mg, 25, 50mg	Up to 200mg/d		
		Indocin SR		75mg	75mg bid		
	Rectal	Indocid	Suppository	100mg	100mg 1-2 times/d		Rectal irritation and occasional bleeding
Ketoprofen	Topical	Oruvail, Powergel Ovuvail Orudis	Gel Tablet Tablet	2.5% 100mg 25–75mg	Apply 2-4 times/d q day 75–225mg/d total		Hypersensitivity reactions
Lornoxicam	Oral	Xefo	Tablet	4mg, 8mg	12mg/d in divided doses	Take with or after food	Gastrointestinal discomfort, nausea, diarrhoea; gastrointestinal bleeding and ulceration; hypersensitivity reactions; headache, dizziness, vertigo, hearing disturbances
Mefenamic acid	Oral	Ponstan Ponstel Ponstan Forte	Capsule Tablet	250mg 250mg 500mg	500mg 3 times/d qid	Take with or after food	Gastrointestinal discomfort, nausea, diarrhoea; gastrointestinal bleeding and ulceration; hypersensitivity reactions; headache, dizziness, vertigo, hearing disturbances

Non-steroidal anti-inflammatory agents (NSAIDs) (continued)

Drug	Format	Trade name	Preparation	Strength	Doses used in arthritis (adult)	Comments	Side effects
Meloxicam	Oral	Mobic	Tablet	7.5mg, 15mg	7.5-15mg/d (elderly 7.5mg/d)	Take with or after food; avoid rectal administration in proctitis or haemorrhoids	Gastrointestinal discomfort, nausea, diarrhoea; gastrointestinal bleeding and ulceration; hypersensitivity reactions; headache, dizziness, vertigo, hearing disturbances
	Rectal	Mobic	Suppository	7.5mg			Rectal irritation and occasional bleeding
Meclofenamate	Oral	Meclomen	Tablet	50-100mg	tid-qid		
Nabumetone	Oral	Relifex	Tablet	500mg	1000-2000mg/d in divided doses	Take with or after food	Gastrointestinal discomfort, nausea, diarrhoea; gastrointestinal bleeding and ulceration; hypersensitivity reactions; headache, dizziness, vertigo, hearing disturbances
		Relafen	Tablet	500, 750mg			
Naproxen	Oral	Naprosyn	Tablet; E/C tablet	250mg, 375mg, 500mg	250-500mg 2 times/d	Take with or after food	Gastrointestinal discomfort, nausea, diarrhoea; gastrointestinal bleeding and ulceration; hypersensitivity reactions; headache, dizziness, vertigo, hearing disturbances
		Naprosyn	Suspension	125mg/5ml	250-500mg 2 times/d		
		Naprosyn S/R	Tablet	500mg	500-1000mg/d		

Non-steroidal anti-inflammatory drugs (NSAIDs) (continued)

Drug	Format	Trade name	Preparation	Strength	Doses used in arthritis (adult)	Comments	Side effects
		Synflex	Tablet	275mg	550mg 2 times/d		
		Napratec	Tablet	500mg (with misoprostol 200mcg)	1 of each tablet taken together 2 times/d	Used as prophylaxis against NSAID-induced gastroduodenal ulceration; contraindicated in pregnant women and women planning a pregnancy	
	Rectal	Naprosyn	Suppository	500mg	500-1000mg/d		Rectal irritation and occasional bleeding
Naproxen Sodium		Anaprox	Tablet	550mg	550-1100mg/d		Gastrointestinal discomfort, nausea, diarrhoea; gastrointestinal bleeding and ulceration; hypersensitivity reactions; headache, dizziness, vertigo, hearing disturbances
Piroxicam	Oral	Feldene (UK & US)	Tablet; capsule	10mg, 20mg	10-30mg/d	Take with or after food	Gastrointestinal discomfort, nausea, diarrhoea; gastrointestinal bleeding and ulceration; hypersensitivity reactions; headache, dizziness, vertigo, hearing disturbances
	Topical	Feldene	Gel	0.5%	Apply 3-4 times/d		Hypersensitivity reactions
	Rectal	Feldene	Suppository	20mg	20mg/d		Rectal irritation and occasional bleeding

Non-steroidal anti-inflammatory agents (NSAIDs) (continued)

Drug	Format	Trade name	Preparation	Strength	Doses used in arthritis (adult)	Comments	Side effects
Sulindac	Oral	Clinoril	Tablet	100mg, 200mg, 150mg, 200mg	200mg 2 times/d 300–400mg/d	Take with or after food	Gastrointestinal discomfort, nausea, diarrhoea; gastrointestinal bleeding and ulceration; hypersensitivity reactions; headache, dizziness, vertigo, hearing disturbances
Tenoxicam	Oral	Mobiflex	Tablet	20mg	20mg/d	Take with or after food	Gastrointestinal discomfort, nausea, diarrhoea; gastrointestinal bleeding and ulceration; hypersensitivity reactions; headache, dizziness, vertigo, hearing disturbances
Tiaprofenic acid	Oral	Surgam	Tablet	200mg, 300mg	600mg/d in divided doses	Contraindicated in patients with urinary tract disorders as severe cystitis has been reported; take with or after food	Gastrointestinal discomfort, nausea, diarrhoea; gastrointestinal bleeding and ulceration; hypersensitivity reactions; headache, dizziness, vertigo, hearing disturbances
		Surgam SA	M/R capsule	300mg	600mg/d		

Cyclo-oxygenase 2 (COX-2) inhibitors

Drug	Format	Trade name	Preparation	Strength	Doses used in arthritis (adult)	Comments	Side effects
Cyclo-oxygenase 2 (COX-2) inhibitors Celecoxib	Oral	Celebrex	Capsule	100mg, 200mg	100-200mg 2 times/d	May be preferred to standard NSAIDs in patients with gastrointestinal ulceration or bleeding or in patients with a high risk of gastrointestinal adverse events; take with or after food	Gastrointestinal discomfort, flatulence, nausea, diarrhoea, gastrointestinal bleeding and ulceration; hypersensitivity reactions; insomnia, headache, dizziness, vertigo, hearing disturbances
Rofecoxib	Oral	Vioxx	Tablet	12.5mg, 25mg	12.5-25mg/d	May be preferred to standard NSAIDs in patients with gastrointestinal ulceration or bleeding or in patients with a high risk of gastrointestinal adverse events; take with or after food	Gastrointestinal discomfort, nausea, diarrhoea, gastrointestinal bleeding and ulceration; hypersensitivity reactions; sleep disturbance, headache, dizziness, vertigo, hearing disturbances, sweating, alopecia
Valdecoxib		Bextra	Tablet	10, 20mg	10-40mg		
Simple analgesia Aspirin	Oral	Generic	Tablet	300mg	300-900mg 4-6h (max. 4000mg/d)	Take with or after food	Gastrointestinal discomfort, gastrointestinal bleeding and ulceration, increased bleeding time, nausea, hearing disturbances, bronchospasm, hypersensitivity reactions
		Caprin	E/C tablet	300mg			
		Nu-Seal	E/C tablet	300mg			

Simple analgesia

Drug	Format	Trade name	Preparation	Strength	Doses used in arthritis (adult)	Comments	Side effects
		Generic	Tablet	400mg (with codeine 8mg)	1-2 tablets 4-6h		Rectal irritation and occasional bleeding
	Rectal	Generic	Suppository	300mg	600-900mg/4h		
Benorilate	Oral	Benoral	Tablet	750mg	4000-8000mg/d in 2-3 divided doses; elderly max. 6g/d	Aspirin-paracetamol ester: 2g benorilate is equivalent to approximately 1.15g aspirin and 970mg paracetamol; take with or after food	Gastrointestinal discomfort, and bleeding, ulceration, increased bleeding time, nausea, hearing disturbances, bronchospasm, hypersensitivity reactions, rashes, blood disorders, acute pancreatitis
		Benoral	Granules	2000mg			
		Benoral	Suspension	5000mg/5ml			
Benzydamine	Topical	Difflam	Cream	3%	Apply 3-6 times/d		Hypersensitivity reactions
Diethylamine salicylate	Topical	Algesal	Cream	10%	Apply 3 times/d		Hypersensitivity reactions
Ethyl nicotinate + hexyl nicotinate + thurfyl salicylate	Topical	Transvasin	Cream	2% + 2% + 14%	Apply 2 times/d		Hypersensitivity reactions
Heparinoid + salicylic acid + thymol	Topical	Movelat	Cream.	0.2% + 2% + 1%	Apply 4 times/d		Hypersensitivity reactions

Simple analgesia (continued)

Drug	Format	Trade name	Preparation	Strength	Doses used in arthritis (adult)	Comments	Side effects
Paracetamol	Oral	Generic	Tablet	500mg	500-1000mg 3-4 times/d		Rashes, blood disorders, acute pancreatitis
		Generic	Suspension	250mg/5ml	1-2 tablets 4 times/d		
		Generic	Tablet	500mg (with codeine 8mg)	1-2 tablets 4 times/d		
		Kapake, Solpadol, Tylex	Tablet, capsule	500mg (with codeine 30mg)			
		Generic	Suppository	250mg	500-1000mg 2 times/d		
Acetaminophen	Oral		Tablet	325, 550mg	up to 1000mg/d in divided dose		Rashes, blood disorders, acute pancreatitis, renal function impairment

Appendix 2 – Useful Addresses and Websites for the GP and Patient

American College of Rheumatology
1800 Century Place, Suite 250,
Atlanta, GA 30345,
USA
Tel: 404 633-3777
Fax: 404 633-1870
Website: www. rheumatology.org

America Juvenile Arthritis Organization
1330 West Peachtree Street
Atlanta, GA 30309,USA
Tel: 800-283-7800
Fax: 404 872 0457

Arthritis Care
18 Stephenson Way
London NW1 2HD
Tel: 020 7916 1500
Fax: 020 7916 1505
Helpline: 0800 289170
Website: www.arthritis care.org.uk

Arthritis Foundation
P.O. Box 7669
Atlanta, GA 30357-0669
USA
Tel: 800 283 7800
Website: www.arthritis.org

Arthritis Research Campaign
PO Box 177
Chesterfield
Derbyshire S41 7TQ
Tel: 01246 558033
Email: info@arc.org.uk
Website: www.arc.org.uk

BackCare
16 Elmtree Road
Teddington
Middlesex TW11 8ST

Tel: 020 8977 5474
Fax: 020 8943 5318
Website: www.backpain.org

British Chiropractic Association
Blagrave House
17 Blagrave Street
Reading RG1 1QB
Tel: 0118 950 5950
Fax: 0118 958 8946
Website: www.chiropractic-uk.co.uk

British Sjögren's Syndrome Association
Unit 1
Manor Workshops
West End
Nailsea BS8 4DD
Tel: 01275 854215
Website:http:/ourworld.compuserve.com/homepages/bssassociation

Chartered Society of Physiotherapy
14 Bedford Row
London WC1R 4ED
Tel: 020 7306 6666
Fax: 020 7306 6611
Email: csp@csphysio.org.uk
Website: www.csp.org.uk

Children's Chronic Arthritis Association (CCAA)
Amber Gate
CityWall Road
Worcester
WR1 2AH
Tel: 01905 745595
Fax: 01905 745703
Website: www.ccaa.org.uk

Dermatomyositis and Polymyositis Support Group
146 Newtown Road
Woolston
Southampton
Hampshire SO19 9HR
Tel: 023 8044 9708

Disabled Living Foundation
380-384 Harrow Road
London W9 2HU
Tel: 020 7289 6111
Helpline: 0845 130 9177
Website: www.dlf.org.uk

Fibromyalgia Association UK
PO Box 206
Stourbridge
West Midlands DY9 8YL
Tel: 01384 820052
Website: www.fmsni.freeserve.c.uk/fmauk.htm

Fibromyalgia Network
PO Box 31750
Tucson
AZ 85751, USA
Website: www.fmnetnews.com

General Osteopathic Council/Osteopathic Information Service
Osteopathy House
176 Tower Bridge Road
London SE1 3LU
Tel: 020 7357 6655
Fax: 020 7357 0011
Website: www.osteopathy.org.uk

Institute for Complementary Medicine
PO Box 194
London SE16 1QZ
Tel: 020 7237 5165
Fax: 020 7237 5175
Website: www.icmedicine.co.uk

Lupus Foundation of America Inc.
1300 Piccard Drive, Suite 200,
Rockville,
MD 20850-4303
USA
Tel: 800 558 0121
Website: www.lupus.org

Lupus UK
St James House
1 Eastern Road
Romford
Essex RM1 3NH
Tel: 01708 731251
Fax: 01708 731252

National Institute of Arthritis & Musculoskeletal & Skin Diseases
National Institutes of Health
1 AMS Circle
Bethesda, Maryland 20892-3675
USA
Tel:301 495 4484
Fax: 301 718 6366
Website: www.niams.nih.gov/.

National Osteoporosis Foundation
1232 22nd Street NW
Washington
DC 20037-1292,
USA
Website: www.nof.org

National Osteoporosis Society
Camerton
Bath BA2 0PJ
Tel: 01761 471771
Helpline: 01761 472721
Website: www.nos.org.uk

Pain Concern (UK)
PO Box 252
Crawley
RH10 3GY
Tel: 01293 552636
Website: www.painconcern.fsnet.co.uk

Patients Association
PO Box 935
Harrow HA1 3YJ
Tel: 020 8423 9111
Fax: 020 8423 9119
Helpline: 020 8423 8999
Website: www. patients-association.com

Raynaud's and Scleroderma Association
112 Crewe Road
Alsager
Cheshire
ST7 2JA
Tel: 01270 872776
Fax: 01270 883556
Website: www.raynauds.demon.co.uk

Royal Association for Disability and Rehabilitation (RADAR)
12 City Forum
250 City Road
London EC1V 8AF
Tel: 020 7250 3222
Fax: 020 7250 0212
Website: www.radar.org.uk

Sjögren's Foundation
8120 Woodmont Avenue, Suite 530
Bethesda
MA, 20814, USA
Tel: 800 475 6473
Website: www.sjogrens.com

Index